ABC of

Sepsis

EDITED BY

Ron Daniels

Chair, Surviving Sepsis Campaign United Kingdom, Consultant in Anaesthesia and Critical Care, Good Hope Hospital, Heart of England NHS Foundation Trust, Birmingham, UK; Fellow, NHS Improvement Faculty

Tim Nutbeam

Specialist Trainee in Emergency Medicine, West Midlands School of Emergency Medicine, Birmingham, UK

KT-102-976

WILEY-BLACKWELL

A John Wiley & Sons, Ltd., Publication

BMJ|Books

This edition first published 2010, © 2010 by Blackwell Publishing Ltd

BMJ Books is an imprint of BMJ Publishing Group Limited, used under licence by Blackwell Publishing which was acquired by John Wiley & Sons in February 2007. Blackwell's publishing programme has been merged with Wiley's global Scientific, Technical and Medical business to form Wiley-Blackwell.

Registered office: John Wiley & Sons Ltd, The Atrium, Southern Gate, Chichester, West Sussex, PO19 8SQ, UK

Editorial offices: 9600 Garsington Road, Oxford, OX4 2DQ, UK
The Atrium, Southern Gate, Chichester, West Sussex, PO19 8SQ, UK
111 River Street, Hoboken, NJ 07030-5774, USA

For details of our global editorial offices, for customer services and for information about how to apply for permission to reuse the copyright material in this book please see our website at www.wiley.com/wiley-blackwell

The right of the author to be identified as the author of this work has been asserted in accordance with the Copyright, Designs and Patents Act 1988.

All rights reserved. No part of this publication may be reproduced, stored in a retrieval system, or transmitted, in any form or by any means, electronic, mechanical, photocopying, recording or otherwise, except as permitted by the UK Copyright, Designs and Patents Act 1988, without the prior permission of the publisher.

Wiley also publishes its books in a variety of electronic formats. Some content that appears in print may not be available in electronic books.

Designations used by companies to distinguish their products are often claimed as trademarks. All brand names and product names used in this book are trade names, service marks, trademarks or registered trademarks of their respective owners. The publisher is not associated with any product or vendor mentioned in this book. This publication is designed to provide accurate and authoritative information in regard to the subject matter covered. It is sold on the understanding that the publisher is not engaged in rendering professional services. If professional advice or other expert assistance is required, the services of a competent professional should be sought.

The contents of this work are intended to further general scientific research, understanding, and discussion only and are not intended and should not be relied upon as recommending or promoting a specific method, diagnosis, or treatment by physicians for any particular patient. The publisher and the author make no representations or warranties with respect to the accuracy or completeness of the contents of this work and specifically disclaim all warranties, including without limitation any implied warranties of fitness for a particular purpose. In view of ongoing research, equipment modifications, changes in governmental regulations, and the constant flow of information relating to the use of medicines, equipment, and devices, the reader is urged to review and evaluate the information provided in the package insert or instructions for each medicine, equipment, or device for, among other things, any changes in the instructions or indication of usage and for added warnings and precautions. Readers should consult with a specialist where appropriate. The fact that an organization or Website is referred to in this work as a citation and/or a potential source of further information does not mean that the author or the publisher endorses the information the organization or Website may provide or recommendations it may make. Further, readers should be aware that Internet Websites listed in this work may have changed or disappeared between when this work was written and when it is read. No warranty may be created or extended by any promotional statements for this work. Neither the publisher nor the author shall be liable for any damages arising herefrom.

Library of Congress Cataloging-in-Publication Data

ABC of sepsis / edited by Ron Daniels, Tim Nutbeam.
      p. ; cm.
   Includes bibliographical references and index.
   ISBN: 978-1-4051-8194-5
   1. Septicemia. I. Daniels, Ron, MD. II. Nutbeam. Tim.
   [DNLM: 1. Sepsis. WC 240 A134 2010]
   RC182.S4A23 2010
   616.9′44--dc22
                          2009018587

A catalogue record for this book is available from the British Library

Set in 9.25/12 Minion by Laserwords Private Limited, Chennai, India
Printed and bound in Singapore
1 2010

ABC of
Sepsis

If found please return to:
Education Centre Library
Wansbeck General Hospital
Woodhorn Lane
Ashington
NE63 9JJ
Tel: 01670 529665

EDUCATION CENTRE LIBRARY

908325

ABC series

An outstanding collection of resources - written by specialists for non-specialists

The *ABC series* contains a wealth of indispensable resources for GPs, GP registrars, junior doctors, doctors in training and all those in primary care

- **Now fully revised and updated**

- **Highly illustrated, informative and practical source of knowledge**

- **An easy-to-use resource, covering the symptoms, investigations, treatment and management of conditions presenting in your day-to-day practice and patient support**

- **Full colour photographs and illustrations aid diagnosis and patient understanding of a condition**

For more information on all books in the *ABC series*, including links to further information, references and links to the latest official guidelines, please visit:

www.abcbookseries.com

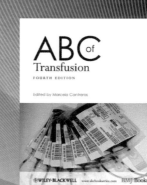

ABC of Transfusion
FOURTH EDITION
Edited by Marcela Contreras

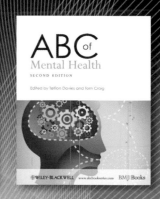

ABC of Mental Health
SECOND EDITION
Edited by Teifion Davies and Tom Craig

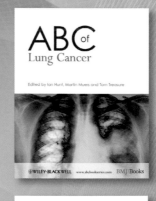

ABC of Lung Cancer
Edited by Ian Hunt, Martin Muers and Tom Treasure

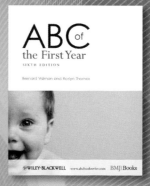

ABC of the First Year
SIXTH EDITION
Bernard Valman and Roslyn Thomas

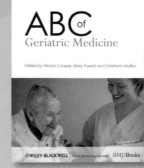

ABC of Geriatric Medicine
Edited by Nicola Cooper, Kirsty Forrest and Graham Mulley

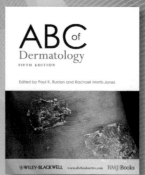

ABC of Dermatology
FIFTH EDITION
Edited by Paul K. Buxton and Rachael Morris-Jones

WILEY-BLACKWELL   BMJ|Books

Contents

Contributors

Sian Abbott

Specialist Registrar in Colorectal Surgery, Good Hope Hospital, Heart of England NHS Foundation Trust, Birmingham, UK

Julian F. Bion

Chair, European Board of Intensive Care Medicine, Professor of Intensive Care Medicine, University of Birmingham, Honorary Consultant in Intensive Care Medicine, University Hospitals Birmingham, Birmingham, UK

Hentie Cilliers

Specialist Registrar in Anaesthesia, West Midlands Deanery, Birmingham, UK

Morgan Cleasby

Consultant Radiologist, Good Hope Hospital, Heart of England NHS Foundation Trust, Birmingham, UK

Ron Daniels

Chair, Surviving Sepsis Campaign United Kingdom, Consultant in Anaesthesia and Critical Care, Good Hope Hospital, Heart of England NHS Foundation Trust, Birmingham, UK; Fellow, NHS Improvement Faculty

Partha De

Consultant Microbiologist, Royal Surrey County Hospital NHS Trust, Guildford, UK

Clare Galvin

Sepsis Nurse Practitioner, Good Hope Hospital, Heart of England NHS Foundation Trust, Birmingham, UK

Nandan Gautam

Consultant in Acute Medicine and Critical Care, University Hospitals Birmingham, Birmingham, UK

Julian Hull

Consultant in Anaesthesia and Critical Care, Good Hope Hospital, Heart of England NHS Foundation Trust, Birmingham, UK

Fiona Lawrence

Professional Development Sister for Critical Care, Good Hope Hospital, Heart of England NHS Foundation Trust, Birmingham, UK

Mitchell M. Levy

Professor of Medicine, The Warren Alpert Medical School of Brown University, Director, Critical Care Services, Rhode Island Hospital, Medical Director, MICU, Rhode Island Hospital, Providence, RI, USA

Georgina McNamara

Sepsis Nurse Practitioner, Good Hope Hospital, Heart of England NHS Foundation Trust, Birmingham, UK

Edwin Mitchell

Specialist Registrar in Anaesthesia and Advanced Intensive Care Medicine Trainee, West Midlands Deanery, Birmingham, UK

Manos Nikoulousis

Specialist Registrar in Haematology, Heart of England NHS Foundation Trust, Birmingham, UK

Tim Nutbeam

Specialist Trainee in Emergency Medicine, West Midlands School of Emergency Medicine, University Hospitals Birmingham, Birmingham, UK

Gavin D. Perkins

Honorary Consultant in Critical Care Medicine, Heart of England NHS Foundation Trust, Co-Director of Research, Intensive Care Society, Associate Clinical Professor in Critical Care and Resuscitation, Warwick University Medical School, Coventry, UK

Gordon D. Rubenfield

Chief, Program in Trauma, Emergency, and Critical Care, Sunnybrook Health Sciences Centre, Professor of Medicine, University of Toronto, Canada

David Stanley

Consultant in Anaesthesia and Intensive Care Medicine, Dudley Group of Hospitals, West Midlands, UK

Jonathan Stewart

Consultant in Colorectal Surgery, Good Hope Hospital, Heart of England NHS Foundation Trust, Birmingham, UK

David R. Thickett

Wellcome Senior Lecturer in Medical Science, University of Birmingham, Honorary Consultant in Respiratory Medicine and Critical Care, University Hospitals Birmingham and Heart of England NHS Foundation Trust, Birmingham, UK

Bill Tunnicliffe

Consultant in Critical Care, University Hospitals Birmingham, Birmingham, UK

Tony Whitehouse

Consultant in Critical Care and Anaesthesia, University Hospitals Birmingham, Birmingham, UK

Preface

Sepsis is a complex condition with a range of aetiologies. Whilst appropriate early intervention has been shown to improve outcome, its recognition and immediate management remain a challenge to healthcare workers.

This book is aimed primarily at doctors, nurses and allied health professionals working in secondary care. It will be most relevant to those working in acute specialities, highlighting the need for prevention where possible, for vigilance, for an immediate response, and for effective collaborative working across disciplines to achieve the best standard of care for these patients.

The diversity and extent of sepsis demands attention by all, however, and those working in primary care may find value too–particularly in causation, pathophysiology and recognition. With increasing resources devoted to pre-hospital emergency care, and widening scopes of practice of paramedical staff, some aspects of immediate diagnostic and therapeutic interventions are becoming increasingly relevant outside the hospital environment.

We hope that you find the *ABC of Sepsis* not only of educational value but also a pragmatic guide to how to manage these patients in your place of work.

Ron Daniels
Tim Nutbeam

CHAPTER 1

Introduction

Mitchell M. Levy

The Warren Alpert Medical School of Brown University, Rhode Island Hospital, Providence, RI, USA

The burden of sepsis on health care is significant. Worldwide, 13 million people become septic each year and 4 million die. In the United States alone, this accounts for approximately 750 000 cases per year, 215 000 resultant deaths, and annual costs of 16.7 billion dollars. Not only is the incidence of severe sepsis higher than that of the major cancers (Figure 1.1) but it has also estimated that in the United Kingdom just under 37 000 deaths are caused annually by the condition – a figure higher than that for lung cancer, or for breast and bowel cancer combined (Figure 1.2). Mortality rates for severe sepsis are 30 to 50%; for septic shock, even higher than 50%. Furthermore, the incidence of sepsis is increasing and will continue to do so as the population ages. Clinicians are challenged to manage this disease in an aging population with multiple co-morbidities, relative immunosuppression and a changing pattern of causative microorganisms.

Defining sepsis

The increasing incidence of sepsis and the high mortality rates associated with the disease have led to global efforts to understand pathophysiology, improve early diagnosis and standardize management. Understanding the spectrum of the disease is important for gauging severity, determining prognosis and developing methods for standardization of care in sepsis. At an international consensus conference in 1991, sepsis was defined as the systemic inflammatory response syndrome (SIRS) with a suspected source of infection.

Organ dysfunction and hypoperfusion abnormalities characterize severe sepsis, while septic shock includes sepsis-induced hypotension despite adequate fluid resuscitation. SIRS and suggested criteria for identifying organ dysfunction and hypoperfusion are discussed further in the next chapter. Although imprecise, these definitions allow for a more uniform approach to clinical trials and the care of the patient with sepsis.

The use of SIRS criteria for the identification of sepsis has been felt by many to be arbitrary and non-specific. In 2001, the terminology was revisited in another consensus conference. At that time, the primary categories of sepsis, severe sepsis and septic shock were confirmed as the best descriptors for the disease process.

The primary change introduced was a more comprehensive list of signs and symptoms that may accompany the disease. This list is described in Chapter 2. In addition, a staging system was proposed for the purpose of incorporating both host factors and response to a particular infectious insult. This concept, termed PIRO (*Predisposition*, *Infection*, *Response*, *Organ dysfunction*) addresses the need to define, diagnose and treat patients with sepsis more precisely, as a variety of evidence-based interventions now exist to improve outcomes in severe sepsis and septic shock. The PIRO model remains hypothetical and is currently being evaluated in several studies.

Pathophysiology – an overview

The pathophysiology of sepsis is dealt with in detail in Chapter 5. Integral to the development of diagnostic and management strategies is an understanding of the interplay between the host's immune, inflammatory and pro-coagulant responses in sepsis. When a given infectious agent invades the host, a non-specific or innate response is triggered via toll-like receptors (TLRs) on immune cells. TLRs are transmembrane proteins with the ability to promote signalling pathways downstream, triggering cytokine release, neutrophil activation and stimulating endothelial cells. This occurs in response to their recognizing a specific pathogen-associated molecule such as lipopolysaccharide. Activation of humoral and cell-mediated – 'adaptive' – immunity follows, with specific B- and T-cell responses and release of both pro- and anti-inflammatory cytokines (some examples of which are listed in Table 1.1) mediated through nuclear factor kappa β. Production of both groups of mediators is significantly increased in patients with severe sepsis.

As adaptive immunity is triggered and the inflammatory cascade of sepsis unfolds, the balance is shifted towards cell death and a state of relative immunosuppression. At this late stage, accelerated lymphocyte apoptosis (programmed cell death) occurs and production of pro-inflammatory mediators may reduce. End-organ dysfunction ensues. Various mediators, including tumour necrosis factor-α (TNF-α) and interleukin 1β (IL-1β), induce nitric oxide production. Not only does this reduce systemic vascular resistance but it also causes myocardial depression and left ventricular dilatation with decreased ejection fraction. The end result of these haemodynamic changes is an elevated cardiac output and generalized vasodilatation. This is often described as 'high-output' shock.

ABC of Sepsis. Edited by Ron Daniels and Tim Nutbeam. © 2010 by Blackwell Publishing, ISBN: 978-1-4501-8194-5.

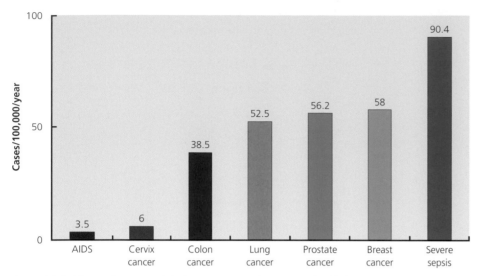

Figure 1.1 Incidence of severe sepsis in Europe. From Davies A. OECD health data 2001. *Intensive Care Medicine* 2001; **27** (suppl): 581.

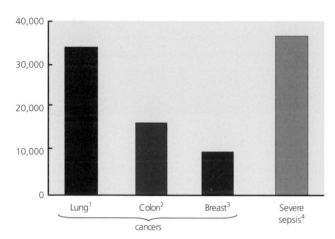

Figure 1.2 Annual mortality from the three biggest cancer killers compared with severe sepsis in the United Kingdom. (1,2,3) Lung, colon, breast cancer data from www.statistics.gov.uk; (4) sepsis data from Intensive Care National Audit Research Centre (2005).

Table 1.1 Some examples of pro-inflammatory and anti-inflammatory cytokines.

Pro-inflammatory
Interleukin 1β (IL-1β)
Interleukin 6
Interleukin 8
Tumour necrosis factor (TNF)-α
Transforming growth factor (TGF)-β

Anti-inflammatory
Interleukin 1 receptor antagonist (IL-1ra)
IL-4
IL-6
IL-10
IL-11
IL-13
Soluble TNF receptors (sTNFr)

As the inflammatory response progresses, myocardial depression becomes more pronounced and may result in a falling cardiac output. Capillary leakage occurs with peripheral and pulmonary oedema that may progress to acute lung injury and acute respiratory distress syndrome (ARDS). A surge in catecholamines, angiotensin II and endothelin causes renal vasoconstriction and increases the risk of renal failure developing. Some of these processes and changes are illustrated in Figure 1.3.

The above changes are accompanied by alterations in the coagulation cascade towards a prothrombotic and antifibrinolytic state mediated by decreased antithrombin III, protein C, protein S and tissue factor pathway inhibitor levels (Figure 1.4). Increased thrombin leads to endothelial and platelet activation. As a result, there is fibrin deposition and microvascular thrombosis which may threaten end organs. The development of disseminated intravascular coagulation in severe sepsis is a predictor of death and the development of multi-organ failure.

Diagnostic challenges in sepsis

Despite advances in our understanding of the disease's mechanisms, it remains difficult to apply these lessons clinically towards early diagnosis and treatment. Addressing this dilemma is paramount given the availability of life-saving interventions, interventions that lose their mortality benefit when delivered late. As the host's initial compensatory mechanisms are overwhelmed and a patient moves through the disease spectrum, tissue beds become hypoxic and injury occurs at the microvascular level. The resultant tissue hypoperfusion, which characterizes severe sepsis and septic shock, can occur despite normal clinical parameters including vital signs and urine output, and may continue following initial resuscitation. Failure to recognize the patient with sepsis and intervene at this stage, prior to or early in the development of organ dysfunction, results in increased morbidity and mortality. Poor outcomes in severe sepsis have been correlated to the development of organ failure on as early as Day 1 following presentation.

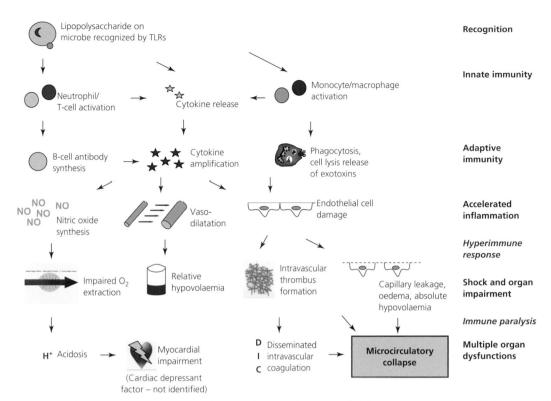

Figure 1.3 Schematic representing stages in the natural course of sepsis and their interactions. Note that multiple organ dysfunctions can also occur in the absence of overt shock through similar mechanisms.

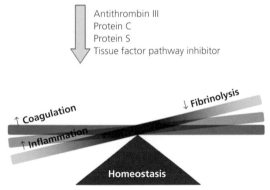

Figure 1.4 Disturbance of the normal balance between pro- and anti-thrombotic tendency seen in severe sepsis. Adapted from Carvalho AC, Freeman NJ. How coagulation defects alter outcome in sepsis. Survival may depend on reversing procoagulant conditions. *Journal of Critical Illness* 1994; **9**: 51–75.

Translating research into clinical practice

Knowledge transfer in medicine remains a difficult and perplexing challenge. All of us, researchers and clinicians alike, have struggled with how and when to incorporate research from the literature into bedside practice. There are numerous obstacles that stand in the way of translating research into bedside practice: first, especially in critical care, clinicians are conservative by nature – which is both good and bad news. The good news is that it means that strategies that have only been partially tested do not regularly get to the bedside and therefore needless harm is prevented for patients.

The bad news is that it takes clinicians a long time to incorporate proven strategies to the bedside.

The second obstacle is that, as busy clinicians, our ability to critically appraise the literature to separate out the mediocre data from the robust randomized control data with good methodology is limited, so there is a lag time between the publication of good data and the implementation of that data.

The publication of several randomized control trials demonstrating mortality reduction with certain interventions in severe sepsis, along with the desire to integrate evidence-based medicine into clinical practice, led to the development of the Surviving Sepsis Campaign (SSC) guidelines. In partnership with the Institute for Healthcare Improvement, the SSC designed the *resuscitation* and *management* bundles in an effort to facilitate knowledge transfer and establish best practice guidelines. Phase III of the SSC is a global quality improvement effort to establish a minimum standard of care for the management of critically ill patients with severe sepsis.

Future directions

The future management of sepsis will most likely involve therapies directed at newer inflammatory targets. Several such molecules are currently under investigation and include, among others: TLR4; the receptor for advance glycation end products (RAGE); and high mobility group box 1 (HMGB-1), a cytokine-like molecule that promotes TNF release from mononuclear cells. HMGB-1 is actively secreted by immunostimulated macrophages and enterocytes and is also released by necrotic but not apoptotic cells. HMGB-1 is now recognized as a pro-inflammatory cytokine.

The use of biomarkers to diagnose, stage and risk assess is another important new field of study. Pro-calcitonin, C-reactive protein, IL-6 and other mediators may be used in combination to develop an 'electrocardiogram' (ECG) of sepsis that may ultimately help guide clinicians to early diagnosis and assist in determining appropriate treatment strategies.

Another important area of ongoing and future research lies in endothelial cells and the microcirculation. Better insight into endothelial cell and microcirculatory dysfunction may direct interventions that will facilitate enhanced restoration of tissue perfusion; a primary pathophysiologic lesion in the inflammatory process that contributes to multi-organ failure and cellular dysfunction in sepsis.

Conclusion

Severe sepsis and septic shock is common and increasing among the critically ill. The opportunity now exists for clinicians to adopt an evidence-based approach to diagnosis and management. Mortality may be reduced by focusing on early diagnosis, targeted management and standardization of the care process.

Further reading

Angus DC, Linde-Zwirble WT, Lidicker J, Clermont G, Carcillo J & Pinsky M. Epidemiology of severe sepsis in the United States: analysis of incidence, outcome, and associated costs of care. *Critical Care Medicine* 2001; **29**: 1303–1310.

Bernard GR, Vincent JL, Laterre PF *et al.* Efficacy and safety of recombinant human activated protein C for severe sepsis. *New England Journal of Medicine* 2001; **344**: 699–709.

Bone RC, Balk RA, Cerra FB *et al.* Definitions for sepsis and organ failure and guidelines for the use of innovative therapies in sepsis. *Chest* 1992; **101**: 1644–1655.

Dellinger RP, Carlet JM, Masur H *et al.* Surviving Sepsis Campaign guidelines for management of severe sepsis and septic shock. *Critical Care Medicine* 2004; **32**: 858–873.

Fourrier F, Chopin C, Goudemand J *et al.* Septic shock, multiple organ failure and disseminated intravascular coagulation. *Chest* 1992; **101**: 816–823.

Gogos CA, Drouou E, Bassaris HP & Skoutelis A. Pro- versus anti-inflammatory cytokine in patients with severe sepsis: a marker for prognosis and future therapeutic options. *Journal of Infectious Diseases* 2000; **181**: 176–180.

Levy MM, Fink MP, Marshall JC *et al.* 2001 SCCM/ESICM/ACCP/ATS/SIS international sepsis definitions conference. *Intensive Care Medicine* 2003; **29**: 530–538.

Levy MM, Macias WL, Vincent JL *et al.* Early changes in organ function predict eventual survival in severe sepsis. *Critical Care Medicine* 2005; **33**: 2194–2201.

Reinhart K, Meisner M & Brunkhorst F. Markers for sepsis diagnosis: what is useful. *Critical Care Clinics* 2006; **22** (3): 503–519.

Rivers E, Nguyen B, Havstad S *et al.* Early goal directed therapy in the treatment of severe sepsis and septic shock. *New England Journal of Medicine* 2001; **345**: 1368–1377.

Russell JA. Management of sepsis. *New England Journal of Medicine* 2006; **355**: 1699–1713.

CHAPTER 2

Defining the Spectrum of Disease

Ron Daniels

Good Hope Hospital, Heart of England NHS Foundation Trust, Birmingham, UK

OVERVIEW

- Consensus international terms including sepsis, severe sepsis and septic shock are used to describe the spectrum of disease
- Precise criteria for the recognition of each stage exist
- Healthcare practitioners need to be aware of the diagnostic tools to facilitate early recognition
- Diagnosis of sepsis is a dynamic and evolving area

Background

A plethora of terms, both medical and colloquial, have been used to describe the inflammatory response to infection – sepsis, septi-caemia, bloodstream poisoning and toxic shock syndrome, to name but a few. As recently as 15 years ago, there existed no international standard in nomenclature in sepsis and no consensus as to precisely when the condition should be diagnosed.

In 1991, a consensus definitions conference headed by the American College of Chest Physicians (ACCP) and Society of Critical Care Medicine (SCCM) was convened to provide guidance on nomenclature and diagnosis. For the first time, healthcare practitioners had a precise set of diagnostic criteria with which to identify the presence of sepsis and an agreement on the terms to be used to describe the process. This, and subsequent revisions, have facilitated not only the recognition and care of these patients but also epidemiological work, observational studies and research into their care.

Nonetheless, the identification of severe sepsis demands vigilance, clinical suspicion and a complex array of observations and laboratory tests. In contrast with the criteria for the identification of acute coronary syndromes (ACS), the recognition of severe sepsis is labour intensive and demanding. Unlike ACS, patients do not present with any one classical clinical picture. Furthermore, a patient may develop or present with severe sepsis as a consequence of any number of conditions, and so all healthcare workers in all disciplines need to be alert.

It should be remembered that a patient with severe sepsis has a mortality of around 35% in the developed world – approximately seven times higher than a patient with ACS. These patients warrant our vigilance and careful evaluation.

Nomenclature

Following the 1991 conference, and having been reaffirmed during a second conference in 2001, a number of terms have become part of healthcare vocabulary. They define the entire spectrum of the condition and are relatively unambiguous. The terms are also valuable in leading the practitioner stepwise through the diagnostic process, each term requiring to be qualified by the former to be of relevance.

Systemic inflammatory response syndrome (SIRS)

The phrase systemic inflammatory response syndrome (SIRS) was first coined during the consensus conference. It describes the inflammatory response seen to a number of triggers, including infection, trauma, burns and pancreatitis. The term is, therefore, non-specific. The physiological and laboratory criteria used to define SIRS have evolved since 1991, and are discussed below.

Inflammation is classically defined as swelling (*tumor*), redness (*rubor*), pain (*dolor*) and heat (*calor*) (Figure 2.1). In the nineteenth century, Virchow added loss of function to the list. At a cellular level,

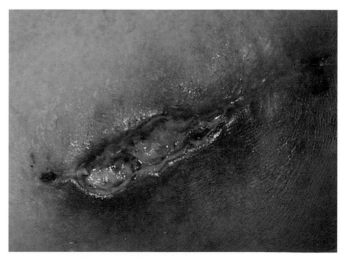

Figure 2.1 Tumor, dolor, rubor and calor.

ABC of Sepsis. Edited by Ron Daniels and Tim Nutbeam. © 2010 by Blackwell Publishing, ISBN: 978-1-4501-8194-5.

the classic changes can be described by vasodilatation, endothelial dysfunction leading to capillary leakage and resultant oedema and the release of cytokines and other inflammatory mediators. These changes are described in more detail in Chapter 5.

At a local level, these changes are beneficial, resulting in a localized hyperaemia to the damaged or infected area bringing oxygen, clotting factors and glucose to effect repair, and humoral and cellular components of the immune system to contain infection. In patients developing severe sepsis, cytokine production appears to be amplified, resulting in a generalized, deleterious vasodilatation, loss of vasomotor control and capillary leakage resulting in relative and actual hypovolaemia and an increase in metabolic demand, which must be met by an increased oxygen delivery to avoid the development of septic shock.

Infection

Infection is perhaps best defined as the presence of micro-organisms in a normally sterile body cavity or fluid (for example, a urinary tract infection), or as an inflammatory response to a micro-organism in a body cavity or fluid which may normally contain micro-organisms (for example, infective colitis).

The majority of organisms causing sepsis are bacterial, as discussed in Chapter 7. A smaller proportion of patients will have fungal infections. The incidence of fungal infections in severe sepsis is rising, with fungi being isolated from 17% of critically ill patients in a recent European study. Fungaemia should be particularly considered in patients with immunocompromise, institutionalized patients and in those with a history of antibiotic use.

Sepsis

The accepted current definition of sepsis is the presence of SIRS criteria in a patient with a new infection.

Severe sepsis

Once sepsis becomes complicated by a dysfunction in one or more organs, this defines severe sepsis. Organs involved may include the lungs (acute lung injury (ALI), hypoxaemia), cardiovascular system (shock, hyperlactataemia), kidneys (oliguria and renal failure), liver (coagulopathy, jaundice, immune paresis), brain (confusion, agitation) and coagulation system (thrombocytopenia, coagulopathy). Criteria for determining organ dysfunction are discussed below.

Septic shock

Septic shock is defined as the persistence of evidence of hypoperfusion despite adequate fluid resuscitation. A patient may qualify as severely septic on the strength of a low blood pressure or high lactate prior to such resuscitation; if these observations persist after fluid challenges this then defines septic shock.

Shock occurs when there is an imbalance between oxygen supply to the tissues and demand (Box 2.1). When this occurs, serum lactate levels rise as a marker of anaerobic respiration. It should be noted that hyperlactataemia is not specific to sepsis. The degree of hyperlactataemia, however, has been shown to be of prognostic

importance, and sequential lactate measurements can help guide fluid resuscitation.

Box 2.1 **Definition of shock**

Tissues are receiving insufficient oxygen and nutrients to satisfy their metabolic needs.

Manifest by one or more of:	
Systolic blood pressure	<90 mmHg
Mean blood pressure	<65 mmHg
Fall in systolic blood pressure	>40 mmHg
Hyperlactataemia, lactate	>4 mmol/l

Clinicians are perhaps more used to considering shock in terms of a patient's blood pressure. Criteria are presented in Box 2.1. There are two potential problems with this rather simplistic approach – patients' normal blood pressures vary widely, particularly with age; and the perfusion of organs depends on blood flow as well as on blood pressure. It is perfectly possible for a patient to have a blood pressure of 180/90 with a cardiac output of less than 2 l/minute. It is sensible, therefore, to consider the blood pressure along with other clinical markers (for example, capillary refill time) and biochemical markers (lactate) in determining the hypoperfused state of shock.

As discussed in Chapter 5, shock in severe sepsis may be multi-factorial. True septic shock is thought of as due to vasodilatation with a reduction in afterload. Remember, however, that a complex syndrome of true and relative hypovolaemia and an element of cardiogenic shock due to unidentified circulating factors are likely to co-exist.

The interrelationship between these terms is summarized in Figure 2.2.

Signs and symptoms of infection

The term 'signs and symptoms of infection' has arisen from the Evaluation for Severe Sepsis Screening Tool developed by the Surviving Sepsis Campaign, and appears from time to time in some literature. The term is appropriate within the context of screening

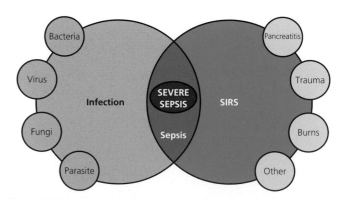

Figure 2.2 Schematic of the interrelationship between systemic inflammatory response syndrome (SIRS), infection and sepsis. AIDS, acquired immune deficiency syndrome.

for sepsis, but is best avoided elsewhere since the criteria (essentially a revised set of SIRS criteria) are not specific to sepsis and are used in the evaluation of the severity of non-infective conditions. This book does not promote the widespread use of this term.

Identifying sepsis

The SIRS criteria originating from the 1991 conference have since been revised. In 2001, a second consensus conference bringing together the SCCM, European Society of Intensive Care Medicine (ESICM), ACCP, American Thoracic Society (ATS) and Surgical Infection Society (SIS) expanded the list of diagnostic criteria for sepsis. This list of diagnostic criteria is presented in Table 2.1.

A stepwise approach to the identification of severe sepsis, adapted from the Surviving Sepsis Campaign's Evaluation for Severe Sepsis Screening Tool, is presented in Figure 2.3. In the United Kingdom, in keeping with the National Institute for Health and Clinical Excellence (NICE) 'Care of the Acutely Ill Patient' guidance, consideration is normally given first to derangements in the patient's physiology.

Table 2.1 Diagnostic criteria for sepsis.

General parameters
Fever (core temperature >38.3°C)
Hypothermia (core temperature <36°C)
Heart rate >90/min or >2 SD above the normal value for age
Tachypnoea: >20/min
Altered mental status
Significant oedema or positive fluid balance
(>20 ml/kg over 24 h)
Hyperglycaemia (plasma glucose >120 mg/dl or 6.7 mmol/l) in the absence of diabetes
Inflammatory parameters
Leukocytosis (white blood cell count >12 000/μl)
Leukopenia (white blood cell count <4000/μl)
Normal white blood cell count with >10% immature forms
Plasma C reactive protein >2 SD above normal value
Plasma calcitonin >2 SD above the normal value
Haemodynamic parameters
Arterial hypotension (SBP <90 mmHg, MAP <65 mmHg, or a decrease in SBP >40 mmHg in adults or <2 SD below normal for age)
Mixed venous oxygen saturation <65%
Central venous oxygen saturation <70%
Cardiac index >3.5 l/min
Organ dysfunction parameters
Arterial hypoxaemia (PaO$_2$/FiO$_2$ <300)
Acute oliguria (urine output <0.5 ml/kg/h for ≥2 h)
Creatinine >176.8 mmol/l
Coagulation abnormalities (INR >1.5 or aPTT >60 s)
Ileus (absent bowel sounds)
Thrombocytopenia (platelet count <100 000/μl)
Hyperbilirubinemia (plasma total bilirubin >34.2 mmol/l)
Tissue perfusion parameters
Hyperlactataemia (>2 mmol/l)
Decreased capillary refill or mottling

SD, standard deviation; SBP, systolic blood pressure; MAP, mean arterial pressure; INR, international normalized ratio; aPTT, activated partial thromboplastin time. Adapted with permission from Levy M, Fink M, Marshall J, *et al. 2001 SCCM/ESICM/ACCP/ATS/SIS International Sepsis Definitions Conference. Intensive Care Medicine* 2003; **29**: 530–538.

IMPORTANT!! If your patient
1. triggers on MEWS
2. has a diagnosis of pneumonia
3. has any other suspicion of infection, apply the:

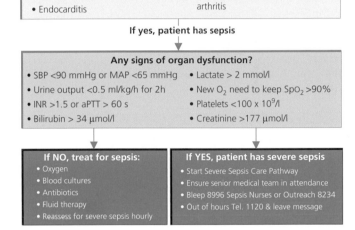

Figure 2.3 Severe Sepsis Screening Tool. MEWS, Modified Early Warning Score; bpm, beats per minute; DM, diabetes mellitus; MAP, mean arterial pressure; aPTT, activated partial thromboplastin time.

Step 1 – Identify SIRS: The recognition of SIRS requires the presence of two or more of the diagnostic criteria (Table 2.2). Revisions over the 1991 criteria include the use of a threshold for hyperthermia of 38.3°C as opposed to 38°C and the addition of acute alterations in mental state and the presence of hyperglycaemia.

Step 2 – Confirm suspicion or evidence of infection: The key point here is that the practitioner must make a thorough evaluation of the patient seeking a likely source of infection. The source does not need to be confirmed – to wait for positive cultures or complex imaging investigations may unnecessarily delay potentially life-saving treatment.

Table 2.2 Diagnostic criteria for systemic inflammatory response syndrome (SIRS).

Temperature >38.3 or <36°C
Heart rate >90/min
Respiratory rate >20/min
White cells <4 or >12 × 10^9/l
Acutely altered mental status
Hyperglycaemia (glucose >6.6 mmol/l) (unless diabetic)

Table 2.3 Possible sources of infection.

Pneumonia, empyema
Urinary tract infection
Acute abdominal infection
Meningitis
Skin/soft tissue infection
Bone/joint infection
Wound infection
Bloodstream catheter infection
Endocarditis
Implantable device infection

Table 2.3 lists possible sources of infection, although this is not exhaustive. Practitioners should guide their history and examination to include or exclude the common sources of infection.

If two or more SIRS criteria are present, and there is a clinically suspected or confirmed source of infection, then this defines the presence of sepsis – a systemic inflammatory response to an infective process.

SIRS + Infection = Sepsis

Step 3 – Evaluate for presence of organ dysfunction: The criteria for determining the presence of organ dysfunction are highlighted in Table 2.4. This demands a complex battery of biochemical, haematological, radiological and physiological investigations and observations. The presence of one criterion for organ dysfunction in the presence of sepsis defines severe sepsis and demands that the patient receive immediate senior medical review.

Sepsis + organ dysfunction = Severe sepsis

The spectrum of sepsis

Sepsis is a continuum. Clearly, the presence of an inflammatory response in the absence of organ dysfunction at one point in time does not infer that the patient will not go on to develop severe sepsis. Patients require close and repeated re-evaluation.

The mortality from sepsis varies according to the presence or absence of organ dysfunction. One large European study, published in 2005, identified hospital mortalities of 26% for patients with

Table 2.4 Diagnostic criteria for organ dysfunction.

SBP <90 mmHg or MAP <65 mmHg
SBP decrease >40 mmHg from baseline
Bilateral pulmonary infiltrates with a new (or increased) oxygen
   requirement to maintain SpO_2 >90%
Bilateral pulmonary infiltrates with PaO_2/FiO_2 ratio <300
Creatinine >176.8 μmol/l or urine output <0.5 ml/kg/h for >2 h
Bilirubin >34.2 μmol/l
Platelet count <100×10⁹/l
Coagulopathy (INR >1.5 or aPTT >60 s)
Lactate >2 mmol/l

SBP, systolic blood pressure; MAP, mean arterial pressure; INR, international normalized ratio; aPTT, activated partial thromboplastin time.

sepsis, 42% for patients with severe sepsis and 61% for patients with septic shock. It is possible that these figures are slightly pessimistic, since data was captured only from intensive care units. Recent unpublished multinational data suggests a mortality rate of 36% from severe sepsis. A combination of shock, renal failure and respiratory failure, not uncommon in severe sepsis, carries a particularly poor prognosis, with a mortality approaching 70%.

When to consider sepsis

A straightforward approach would be to evaluate for the presence of sepsis in any patient admitted with a suspicion of infection.

This is unfortunately rather simplistic in that it does not take account of the dynamic nature of the condition. As teams of nurses and clinicians caring for patients, we are increasingly using physiological 'track and trigger' warning systems to detect deterioration and severity of disease. Such systems lend well to the diagnosis of severe sepsis. It is good practice to apply a 'screening tool' for severe sepsis whenever one of these systems is triggered in a patient. Similarly, if a patient deteriorates unexpectedly or fails to improve as expected, particularly in the presence of risk factors such as indwelling devices or recent surgery, it is good practice to evaluate for severe sepsis.

Future strategies

It is tempting to think that we may, in the future, be able to identify sepsis using a more straightforward approach. Teams are attempting to identify an 'ECG' of markers for sepsis. Promising markers include procalcitonin, cytokines including interleukin 6, adrenomedullin and soluble endothelial/leukocyte adhesion molecules. It is likely that a combination of factors will be required and that sensitivity and specificity will not be sufficiently high to replace clinical assessment.

The PIRO system is discussed in Chapter 1. It may provide a means in the future to more accurately delineate differences between patients with sepsis, but requires further development and evaluation. Broadly, it examines patients across four domains: 'P' for Predisposition, or at-risk factors; 'I' for Infection or infective insult and magnitude; 'R' for Response of the host to that insult and 'O' for Organ dysfunction. Conceptually, it is attractive in that patients could be graded for severity in each domain, analogous to the tumour-node-metastasis (TNM) system in cancer staging.

Conclusion

Patients in hospitals have multiple risk factors for the development of severe sepsis. They are ill, will usually have indwelling devices such as intravenous cannulae, and are exposed to a wide range of bacteria, some of which may have developed antibiotic resistance. They may be, or have been, treated with antimicrobial drugs themselves, increasing the risk of colonization with organisms resistant to multiple antibiotics. They may be elderly or very young, and some will be immunocompromized either as a result of their acute illness, because of drugs administered to them in the course of their treatment, or through congenital or acquired immunodeficiencies.

Healthcare workers need to recognize that each and every patient in hospital is at risk of severe sepsis. An infective cause must be considered whenever a patient presents with acutely altered physiology, deteriorates unexpectedly during treatment for another condition or simply fails to improve as expected.

Severe sepsis is recognized as a systemic response to an infection, resulting in both physiological disturbance and organ dysfunction (including shock). A tool to recognize the presence of sepsis and severe sepsis according to international definitions is presented, and should be applied whenever an infection is likely.

Healthcare professionals can therefore precisely determine the presence or absence of severe sepsis for an individual patient. As we shall discover, the early identification and immediate management of these patients is essential if we are to improve outcome.

Further reading

Angus DC, Burgner D, Wunderink R *et al*. The PIRO concept: P is for predisposition. *Critical Care* 2003; **7**: 248–251.

Bone RC, Balk R, Cerra FB *et al*. ACCP/SCCM Consensus Conference: Definitions for sepsis and organ failure and guidelines for use of innovative therapies in sepsis. *Chest* 1992; **101**: 1644–1655.

Lever A & Mackenzie I. Sepsis: definition, epidemiology, and diagnosis. *British Medical Journal* 2007; **335**: 879–883.

Levy MM, Fink MP, Marshall JC *et al*. 2001 SCCM/ESICM/ACCP/ATS/SIS~ international sepsis definitions conference. *Critical Care Medicine* 2003; **31**: 1250–1256.

Marik PE. Editorial: definition of sepsis: not quite time to dump SIRS? *Critical Care Medicine* 2002; **30** (3): 706–708.

CHAPTER 3

Identifying the Patient with Sepsis

Ron Daniels

Good Hope Hospital, Heart of England NHS Foundation Trust, Birmingham, UK

OVERVIEW

- The importance of basic clinical assessment should not be overlooked

- Tools such as track-and-trigger warning scores are useful in identifying critically ill patients

- A Sepsis/Severe Sepsis Screening Tool will help confirm a clinical suspicion of sepsis

- Effective communication of clinical findings is vital to ensure that appropriate care is delivered in a timely fashion

Introduction

The reliable recognition of sepsis, in order to initiate appropriate treatments in a timely fashion, is a challenge for all health care organizations. Patients are admitted under all specialities and with a wide variety of modes of presentation. Some presentations point directly to the causative pathology – for example, a patient presenting with dyspnoea and a productive cough would naturally be suspected to have pneumonia. Others are more non-specific: consider an elderly patient arriving after having collapsed at home. The differential diagnosis will include a cerebral event, acute dysrhythmia or myocardial infarction, an endocrine or metabolic crisis and drug toxicity in addition to sepsis.

A number of patients will present with a condition that itself requires immediate and specific resuscitation – for example, a patient with diabetic keto-acidosis will require rapid fluid resuscitation and correction of hyperglycaemia with attention to electrolyte disturbance. In this instance, the resuscitation may distract from both the underlying infective process and the additional aspects of resuscitation needed in the context of severe sepsis.

Similarly, the time course of the disease varies widely. Patients with meningococcal or pneumococcal septicaemia, for example, tend to present in extremis, frequently with shock, acidosis and oliguria. They may have been well enough to have worked the previous day. Other conditions have a more insidious onset, with the patient describing a protracted illness with some mild influenza-like

ABC of Sepsis. Edited by Ron Daniels and Tim Nutbeam. © 2010 by Blackwell Publishing, ISBN: 978-1-4501-8194-5.

symptoms that have worsened over days or weeks. Examples include pneumonia due to atypical organisms, some urinary tract infections and osteomyelitis.

The conditions causing sepsis and their relative frequency are shown in Box 3.1.

Box 3.1 **Causes of severe sepsis and their relative frequencies**

Pneumonia	50–60%
Intra-abdominal	20–25%
Urinary tract infection	7–10%
Soft tissue, bone, joint	5–10%
Endocarditis	<5%
Meningitis	<5%

Recognition of severe sepsis

The key to the reliable recognition of severe sepsis is to have a high index of suspicion. This is important for an individual healthcare worker, but organizations and departments will also benefit from developing a culture of suspicion of severe infection.

The consensus definitions criteria introduced in Chapter 2 provide a basis for Sepsis and Severe Sepsis Screening Tools in use in a number of organizations around the world. An example of such a tool is given in Figure 3.1. The complexity of current criteria for identifying sepsis and severe sepsis means that such tools are invaluable, whether as visual prompts in prominent locations or as part of admission or ongoing evaluation documentation.

A screening tool will only be effective if it is frequently, appropriately and accurately used. Staff need to be aware, if the tool is used as an 'opt in' document rather than universally, of when to consider its use. One approach is to apply the screening tool whenever a patient is admitted with, or later develops, a diagnosis or clinical suspicion of infection. As indicated above, it is easier to identify some infections than others, so the use of this approach alone may lead to a delay in diagnosis for many patients. It is sensible to combine a diagnosis-based approach like this with a physiology-based approach as discussed below.

A third strategy relies on the clinical experience of a nurse, doctor or allied health professional – the 'end of the bed' test. If the clinical condition of a patient does not improve over time as

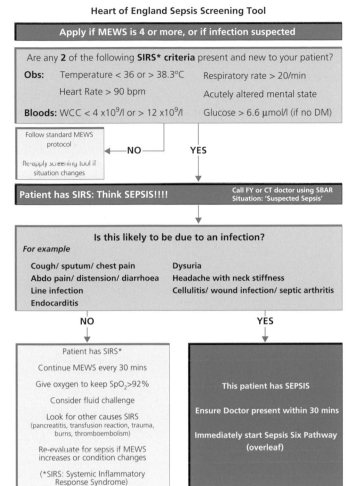

Heart of England Sepsis Screening Tool

Apply if MEWS is 4 or more, or if infection suspected

Are any **2** of the following **SIRS* criteria** present and new to your patient?

Obs: Temperature < 36 or > 38.3°C   Respiratory rate > 20/min

Heart Rate > 90 bpm   Acutely altered mental state

Bloods: WCC < 4 x10⁹/l or > 12 x10⁹/l   Glucose > 6.6 µmol/l (if no DM)

Follow standard MEWS protocol / Re-apply screening tool if situation changes ← NO   YES

Patient has SIRS: Think SEPSIS!!!!   Call FY or CT doctor using SBAR Situation: 'Suspected Sepsis'

Is this likely to be due to an infection?

For example

Cough/ sputum/ chest pain   Dysuria
Abdo pain/ distension/ diarrhoea   Headache with neck stiffness
Line infection   Cellulitis/ wound infection/ septic arthritis
Endocarditis

NO   YES

Patient has SIRS*

Continue MEWS every 30 mins

Give oxygen to keep SpO₂>92%

Consider fluid challenge

Look for other causes SIRS
(pancreatitis, transfusion reaction, trauma, burns, thromboembolism)

Re-evaluate for sepsis if MEWS increases or condition changes

(*SIRS: Systemic Inflammatory Response Syndrome)

This patient has SEPSIS

Ensure Doctor present within 30 mins

Immediately start Sepsis Six Pathway (overleaf)

Figure 3.1 Sepsis Screening Tool. MEWS, Modified Early Warning Score; bpm, beats per minute; DM, diabetes mellitus; WCC, white cell count.

Box 3.2 illustrates how an aggregate MEWS score is calculated from a set of observations.

Box 3.2 **Calculation of an aggregated track-and-trigger score**

Score	3	2	1	0	1	2	3
Respiratory rate		<8		9–19	20–22	23–30	>30
SpO₂ %	<88	88–89	90–95	≥96			
Heart rate	<40	40–49	50–89	90–109	110–129		>130
Systolic BP	<70	70–79	80–99	100–199		>200	
Urine output	Nil	<20 ml/hr	<30 ml/hr				
Central nervous system (CNS)		Confused		Alert	Voice	Pain	Unresponsive
Temperature		<35	35–35.9	36.0–37.2	37.3–38.2	≥38.3	

Example

Respiratory rate	20	Score 1
SpO₂	97%	0
Heart rate	110	1
Systolic BP	85 mmHg	1
Urine output (Just admitted)	Unknown	0
CNS	Alert	0
Temperature	35°C	1
Total		**4**

Mandates assessment by Critical Care Outreach and medical team within 30 minutes.

Aggregate scoring systems are recommended in the United Kingdom by the National Institute for Health and Clinical Excellence, and supported by the National Outreach Forum (NOrF). The MEWS system has been validated as a predictor of outcome in acute medical admissions in one large study. These systems can provide a useful stimulus to apply a Sepsis/Severe Sepsis Screening Tool. A prompt to do this is integrated into the track-and-trigger system in many hospitals. Audit has demonstrated that, in acute hospitals in the United Kingdom with a mixed caseload, sepsis and severe sepsis account for around half of all episodes of MEWS triggers. It is, therefore, sensible to apply a screening tool whenever the track-and-trigger system prompts a referral to the emergency team.

expected, or deteriorates unexpectedly, then sepsis should be considered as a common cause of deterioration. A classic example is the patient who remains intolerant of oral intake some days following a laparotomy for bowel resection with anastomosis. This would usually be regarded as unusual, and should alert the team to seek an intra-abdominal collection of fluid or an anastomotic leak.

Track-and-trigger scoring systems

Systems such as the Early Warning Score (EWS) or modified versions (Modified Early Warning Score (MEWS)), Patient at Risk Scores (PARS) and Medical Emergency Team (MET) calling criteria are based on the identification of physiological derangement from the normal range. Systems vary, but commonly aggregate scores for individual parameters according to the severity of their abnormality. When the scores for each observation added together exceed a 'trigger point', a response is required. This may be a call to the emergency medical team or another member of the same team. Simpler systems 'code' observations using colour and prompt response when any single observation deviates significantly from its normal range.

Clinical assessment of the patient

It is sensible to adopt a standardized, systematic approach to the assessment of any deteriorating or critically ill patient, including those with sepsis and severe sepsis. Clinical signs are readily and appropriately assessed using the ABCDE system. The underlying pathophysiology is discussed in more detail in Chapter 5.

Airway

An assessment should be made of the patency of the patient's airway, particularly if the patient's conscious level is reduced. Clearly, if the patient is awake and talking, there is little likelihood of an airway problem. Hypoperfusion of the brain in septic shock may precipitate the loss of an airway.

Look: The mouth should be examined to determine the presence of excessive secretions, vomitus or solid matter. Clinical signs suggesting partial obstruction include tracheal tug, nasal flaring, recession of the intercostal muscles and 'see-saw' respiration.

Listen: Abnormal inspiratory noises such as stridor (indicating partial obstruction) and gurgling (indicating secretions or vomitus in the mouth) should be sought.

Feel: The back of the practitioner's hand placed close to the patient's mouth and nose can detect the movement of warm exhaled air.

If an airway problem is identified, it should be rectified immediately in line with appropriate life support guidelines. Consideration should be given to the need for oxygen therapy even in the absence of an identifiable airway problem. Patients with severe sepsis will benefit from high-flow oxygen therapy.

Breathing

The body's demand for oxygen rises in severe sepsis. As demand outstrips supply, lactic acidosis occurs. These processes combine to elevate the respiratory rate. If the underlying condition is pneumonia, if abdominal distension or pain is causing splinting of the diaphragm, or if shock has resulted in hypoperfusion of the lungs, hypoxaemia may result.

Look: The presence of central cyanosis suggests hypoxaemia. The patient's respiratory rate, depth and pattern should be evaluated in addition to any asymmetry of chest movement. The use of accessory muscles should alert the clinician to impending fatigue and a possible need for ventilation.

Listen: Abnormal sounds include expiratory wheezes, suggesting obstruction of the lower airways; and crepitations, suggestive of secretions, pulmonary oedema or a consolidation. Percussion of the chest may help differentiate between pleural effusions and consolidation when breath sounds are diminished in one area. The silent chest is an emergency, indicating impending respiratory arrest.

Feel: Occasionally, crepitations may be palpable on the chest surface.

If a respiratory problem is identified, attention should be given to oxygen therapy and to the possible need for bronchodilators

and physiotherapy. The response to therapy should be assessed repeatedly. Pulse oximetry is mandatory, and arterial blood gases and a chest X-ray may be helpful.

Circulation

The impact of sepsis on the circulation is multifactorial, as discussed in Chapter 5. Attention should be paid to clinical signs of adequacy of blood flow and to the heart rhythm. This is of equal importance to blood pressure measurement.

Look: Attention should be paid to the colour of the skin, particularly peripherally. Pallor is suggestive of hypoperfusion and may suggest a low cardiac output state. Mottled skin indicates imminent or established circulatory collapse.

Listen: If experienced in doing so, the heart sounds should be auscultated, particularly seeking a murmur. If new to the patient, this may be suggestive of subacute bacterial endocarditis as the source of sepsis, and mandates an urgent echocardiogram.

Feel: The back of the hand can be used to assess peripheral skin temperature. In decompensated sepsis, where the cardiac output begins to fall, the peripheries may appear cool. There may be a line of demarcation where warm skin gives way to cool. The capillary refill time is an underperformed and useful test of perfusion. Pressure should be applied over the pulp of the thumb for 5 seconds and then released (Figure 3.2). Colour will normally return within 2 seconds. Sequential capillary refill tests are a useful adjunct in guiding fluid resuscitation.
The heart rate and rhythm should be assessed by palpation of peripheral pulses. In shock, more central pulses only may be palpable.

Clinical evaluation of the cardiovascular system will be supplemented by the measurement of blood pressure, by a 12-lead electrocardiogram (ECG) to identify any dysrhythmias, and by obtaining a lactate measurement to assess the adequacy of global tissue perfusion.

Disability

Reduced cerebral perfusion, and the resultant variable agitation, confusion and depressed conscious levels this can produce, is common in sepsis. Fluid resuscitation can restore cerebral function.

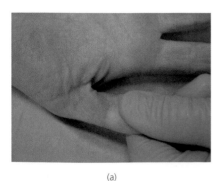
(a)

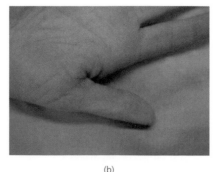
(b)

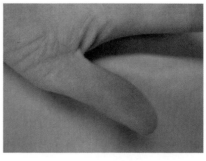
(c)

Figure 3.2 Capillary refill assessment. (a) Press on the pulp of the thumb for 5 seconds. (b) Immediately on removing pressure, the tissue will be blanched. (c) Colour should return within 2 seconds.

It is important to remember to measure the blood glucose, since hypoglycaemia can also produce any of these signs and is readily correctable. Signs of meningism – photophobia, neck stiffness and a positive Kernig's sign – should be sought. If there is clinical suspicion of meningitis, senior help should urgently be sought and cerebral imaging and lumbar puncture urgently arranged. Early administration of antibiotics is vital in this context.

The conscious level can be quickly assessed and communicated using the AVPU Scale:

A	**A**lert
V	Responds to **V**oice
P	Responds to **P**ain
U	**U**nresponsive

A score of P or U correlates well with a Glasgow Coma Score of 7 or less, indicating the need for urgent airway protection. The Glasgow Coma Score is illustrated in Box 3.3. If the conscious level is reduced or is deteriorating, particularly in the presence of localizing neurological signs, urgent imaging is required.

Box 3.3 **The Glasgow Coma Score (minimum score 3, maximum 15)**

Best motor response (assess 'best' response from any limb)
1. No response to pain
2. Extensor posturing to pain
3. Abnormal flexor response to pain
4. Withdraws to pain
5. Localizing response to pain
6. Obeying command

Best Verbal Response (record best level of speech)
1. None
2. Incomprehensible speech
3. Inappropriate speech
4. Confused conversation
5. Orientated

Eye Opening
1. No eye opening
2. Eye opening in response to pain
3. Eye opening in response to any speech
4. Spontaneous eye opening

Exposure

The patient should be examined from head to toe seeking the source of sepsis. Particular attention should be paid at this point to the abdomen – a tense, distended abdomen with absent bowel sounds should be assessed immediately by a senior surgeon. Limbs, and especially the joints, should be examined carefully for swelling and erythema suggestive of underlying septic arthritis or osteomyelitis.

Any drain or indwelling device should be noted, evaluated for signs of infection at the insertion site and their output assessed if appropriate. Consideration should be given to removal of any indwelling device, particularly if the insertion site appears inflamed.

Consideration should be given to the patient's dignity during this assessment, and it should be recognized that exposure can cause rapid temperature loss. It is useful to measure core and peripheral temperatures and to monitor the difference – as the circulation is restored during resuscitation the difference should reduce.

Investigations

These are covered in detail in other chapters. Once a clinical assessment has been completed, or if it highlights the need for urgent investigation, tests should be arranged without delay.

All patients with potential sepsis should have blood cultures taken, preferably from at least two sites. Consideration should be given to urine, sputum and cerebrospinal fluid cultures; and collections of pus identified should be aspirated percutaneously or drained surgically and samples sent.

All patients should have their serum lactate measured. In cases of 'covert' or 'cryptic' septic shock, where the blood pressure is normal, an elevated lactate can give an early indication of the need for rapid fluid resuscitation. It is also useful to know the haemoglobin concentration, white blood cell count and differential, platelet count, electrolyte levels and biochemical markers of hepatic enzymes and renal function. A coagulation screen may help identify early disseminated intravascular coagulopathy (DIC).

The source of sepsis needs identifying early. In sepsis of unknown origin, a chest X-ray should be ordered. An abdominal ultrasound examination may be helpful. The clinical examination will guide other, more specific imaging investigations.

If imaging supported by clinical assessment is suggestive of a collection of potentially infected fluid, such as a deep abscess, immediate attention should be given to percutaneous or surgical drainage.

Communication

Most organizations will have a clear communications policy in the care of the critically ill. The practitioner should be aware of sources of immediate expert advice. Examples include Critical Care Outreach, the Medical Emergency Team, and the immediate seniors within the admitting team. In most cases of septic shock, Critical Care should be contacted urgently.

In the United Kingdom, a number of studies have demonstrated that failure to escalate a complex case to senior colleagues, and failure to refer appropriately, contribute to a high percentage of avoidable deaths in hospitals. As discussed in Chapter 1, sepsis carries a high mortality. In the context of severe sepsis, there is no excuse for the patient not to be assessed by senior medical staff as soon as possible, and for the majority of cases within the first hour of the condition being recognized.

SBAR

Developed by the U.S. Navy Nuclear Submarine Service, SBAR – **S**ituation, **B**ackground, **A**ssessment, **R**ecommendation – is directly applicable as a communications tool to many aspects of healthcare delivery, and nowhere more so than in the care of the critically ill patient. An example of SBAR used in a telephone referral is given in Box 3.4.

Box 3.4 Example of SBAR use in a clinical situation

Situation

'I have a 65-year-old lady in the Emergency Department with septic shock secondary to an acute abdomen probably secondary to a perforated viscus'.

Background

'She has a history of diverticular disease and she was admitted for 5 days with acute diverticulitis last month. This settled with conservative treatment. She became unwell again last week with acute colicky abdominal pain and constipation, and is now vomiting and unable to tolerate oral intake. She is previously fit and healthy and on no regular medication'.

Assessment

'She is acutely distressed and looks unwell.

A She is maintaining her airway
B Her respiratory rate is 20. She is adequately oxygenated with a saturation of 97% on 60% inspired oxygen.
C Her peripheries are cool with a cap refill time of 6 seconds.
   Following 2 litres of Hartmann's stat, she remains tachycardic with a heart rate of 110 and a blood pressure of 85/40. Her lactate was initially 6 and is now 5 mmol/l.
D She is fully conscious and alert. Her blood glucose is slightly elevated.
E Her temperature is 35°C. Her abdomen is distended and tense with absent bowel sounds.

   Her arterial blood gases (ABGs) show a metabolic acidosis. A portable chest X-ray demonstrates air under the diaphragm. I have requested bloods including cultures and am awaiting results.'

Recommendation

'I would like you to come and assess this lady urgently as I think she may need a laparotomy for perforated viscus. I am continuing fluid resuscitation and have started antibiotics according to the protocol. I have also requested Critical Care to attend'.

Conclusion

Clinical assessment of all potentially critically ill patients is vital. In a culture of diagnosis-based medicine, where practitioners seek to 'label' a condition, it is sometimes easy to ignore physiological alterations that may herald systemic sequelae of a primary condition. Clinicians, nurses and allied health professionals should adopt a high index of suspicion of sepsis and actively seek an infective cause in the acutely ill. Tools such as track-and-trigger physiological warning systems can help identify patients at risk, and a Sepsis/Severe Sepsis Screening Tool can help identify patients with these conditions. Effective communication and escalation of care are vital to ensure that the best care is delivered by the right people at the right time.

Further reading

Goldhill DR, McNarry AF, Mandersloot G & McGinley A. A physiologically-based early warning score for ward patients: the association between score and outcome. *Anaesthesia* 2005; **60** (6): 547–553.

Helmreich RL. On error management: lessons from aviation. *British Medical Journal* 2000; **320** (7237): 781–785.

Pope BB, Rodzen L & Spross G. Raising the bar with SBAR: How better communication improves patient outcomes. *Nursing* 2008; **38** (3): 41–3.

Resuscitation Council (UK). *A Systematic Approach to the Acutely Ill Patient*, June 2005. Online at www.resus.org.uk.

Subbe C, Kruger M, Rutherford P & Gemmel L. Validation of a modified early warning score in medical admissions. *QJM: An International Journal of Medicine* 2001; **94**: 521–526.

CHAPTER 4

Serious Complications of Sepsis

Hentie Cilliers[1], Tony Whitehouse[2] and Bill Tunnicliffe[2]

[1]West Midlands Deanery, Birmingham, UK
[2]University Hospitals Birmingham, Birmingham, UK

OVERVIEW

- For most patients, serious sequelae can be avoided with early identification and appropriate early intervention
- Immediate sequelae relate to the acute inflammatory process, with relative hypoperfusion, damage due to microthrombi and disrupted capillary basement membranes
- Organ support at a Critical Care level is frequently required in the acute phase
- Most organ dysfunction will ultimately resolve if supported appropriately
- A minority of patients will suffer permanent sequelae, for example, from digital ischaemia, pulmonary fibrosis and psychological disturbances

Introduction

Mortality from severe sepsis and septic shock remains high. As has been outlined in previous chapters, the spectrum of sepsis can develop from relatively mild systemic inflammatory response syndrome (SIRS) through to full-blown multi-organ dysfunction syndrome (MODS) (Figure 4.1). This disease continuum is characterized by increasing mortality as shown in Figure 4.2.

Sepsis is defined as a suspected or proven infection in the presence of two or more of the SIRS criteria. Therefore, complications and serious sequelae of sepsis in simple terms include severe sepsis, septic shock and MODS.

Treated early, SIRS is reversible for the majority of patients and not associated with long-term adverse outcomes. Indeed, many aspects of MODS may be completely reversible with time.

The most obvious serious consequence of sepsis is death. Traditionally, mortality rates of severe sepsis have been quoted between 30 and 50%. These data are likely to be skewed by a Critical Care bias and the true mortality for all patients satisfying the diagnostic criteria may be lower. Critical Care Outreach, the sepsis care bundles and new therapies may contribute to a lower overall mortality, and this will vary depending on the patient's co-morbidities, genetic predisposition and the causative organism.

ABC of Sepsis. Edited by Ron Daniels and Tim Nutbeam. © 2010 by Blackwell Publishing, ISBN: 978-1-4501-8194-5.

Untreated, sepsis may lead to severe physiological and biochemical disruption. Although the early stages of sepsis are normally characterized by pyrexia, vasodilatation and a hyperdynamic circulation, this can progress (very rapidly with some causative organisms) to a patient who is hypothermic, vasoconstricted and in a low cardiac output state.

Cardiovascular

The cardiovascular changes associated with sepsis lead to altered blood flow to organs as well as within organs. A reduced intravascular volume due to dilatation of venous capacitance and arteriolar vessels compounded by an increase in endothelial permeability can lead to a profound drop in blood pressure and cardiac output (septic shock). This leads to peripheral hypoperfusion, and the resulting increase in serum lactic acid may act as a myocardial depressant. A vicious circle ensues due to the reduction in cardiac output.

A fall in diastolic pressure may reduce flow distal to atheromatous disease and cause infarction of the tissue beyond. Furthermore, the increase in cardiac output increases cardiac work, which may cause compromise in a patient with ischaemic heart disease.

Biventricular dilatation and reduced ejection fraction are present in most patients with sepsis syndromes. Myocardial depression exists despite a fluid resuscitation-dependent hyperdynamic state that typically persists in patients with septic shock until death or recovery. Cardiac function usually recovers within 7–10 days in survivors. Myocardial dysfunction is almost certainly not due to myocardial hypoperfusion but due to circulating depressant factors, possibly including the cytokines tumour necrosis factor and interleukin (IL)-1β.

Respiratory

Lung dysfunction (respiratory failure) is one of the most common complications of severe sepsis, developing in 18–38% of patients. It is initially an indirect process, but secondary infections and trauma from mechanical ventilation can exacerbate the lung injury.

Pathologically, there is diffuse alveolar damage (DAD) caused by an intra- and perivascular inflammatory response initiated by the presence of endotoxins in the blood. The cycle of injury and

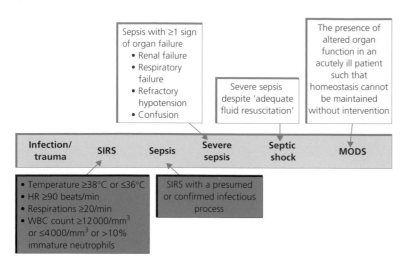

Figure 4.1 Bone's criteria for the recognition of severe sepsis and the spectrum of the disease. SIRS, systemic inflammatory response syndrome; MODS, multi-organ dysfunction syndrome; HR, heart rate; WBC, white blood cell.

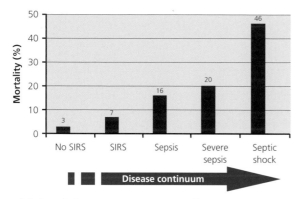

Figure 4.2 A survival spectrum. SIRS, systemic inflammatory response syndrome. Rangel-Frausto MS *et al*. The natural history of the systemic inflammatory response syndrome (SIRS). A prospective study. *The journal of the American Medical Association* 1995; **273** (2): 117–123.

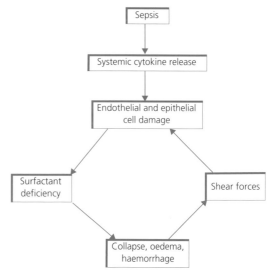

Figure 4.3 Sequence of events that lead to, and may perpetuate, lung damage in sepsis syndromes.

damage is shown in Figure 4.3. DAD goes through stages termed the exudative, regenerative and repair phases. The inflammatory process disrupts the alveolar wall and allows infiltration of neutrophils. In the exudative phase, proteinaceous oedema fluid leaks into the alveolae and there is damage of type 1 epithelial cells. Histologically, this is often termed 'shock lung' and is characterized by:

• alveolar collapse, haemorrhage and oedema;
• hyaline membrane formation on the epithelial surface of respiratory bronchioles and alveolar ducts: this comprises fibrin and necrotic epithelial cells;
• variable neutrophil accumulation in alveolar capillaries.

If left untreated, patients can develop severe pulmonary oedema (despite low central venous pressure) and progressive impairment of diffusion of oxygen and carbon dioxide. This is then called the acute respiratory distress syndrome (ARDS) and unless the intra-alveolar exudate is reduced by positive pressure airway support, the resulting ventilation/perfusion mismatch (effectively right-to-left shunting) causes severe hypoxaemia and presents significant challenges in oxygenation.

The regenerative phase allows healing of the lung either to its normal structure or progresses to fibrosis via the repair phase. Type 2 epithelial cells proliferate to replace the lost type 1 epithelium; they may be large and elongated, resembling macrophages in the airways. The epithelium may regrow beneath the hyaline membrane, which is sloughed off, or over the membrane, in which case it becomes incorporated into the alveolar wall and is a mechanism for the development of interstitial fibrosis. In capillaries, the endothelial repair may be accompanied by local thrombosis, organization and local vascular remodelling. Along with progressive interstitial thickening, the alveolar exudate organizes. This fibrosis (Figure 4.4) can happen within weeks although some authors believe that it may start very early in the course of acute lung injury and is the rationale behind studies of the use of steroids in ARDS.

Through interstitial fibrosis, therefore, patients can suffer permanent functional restrictions and limitations of lifestyle following successful treatment of severe sepsis.

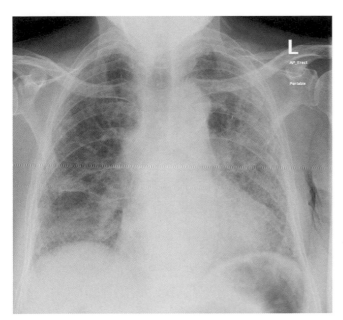

Figure 4.4 Pulmonary fibrosis as a late complication of sepsis-induced lung injury.

Renal

Renal failure often accompanies sepsis, with an incidence of 23% in cases of severe sepsis. The mortality of sepsis complicated by acute renal failure can be as high as 70%. Acute tubular necrosis is caused by hypotension, intravascular dehydration, release of cytokines and renal vasoconstriction. However, as discussed below, renal failure may occur in the absence of acute tubular necrosis. Renal replacement therapies (RRTs) like continuous veno-venous haemofiltration (Figure 4.5) and haemodialysis improve the biochemical status but have not been shown convincingly to contribute to a reduction in mortality. A number of units use aggressive continuous veno-venous haemofiltration (CVVH) to remove the increased amount of inflammatory products in an attempt to halt the progression of sepsis, although this practice is not supported by a large body of evidence.

Sepsis-induced acute renal impairment in previously healthy individuals often reveals little significant histological change on renal biopsy (even in those patients who die from sepsis), and recovery of renal function from complete anuria and biochemical derangement is possible. This may, however, take several months despite early resolution of systemic inflammation and restoration of a normal circulatory profile. Renal failure is usually reversible to such a degree that most patients become independent of RRT; an audit of Scottish intensive care units (ICUs) in 2001 showed the percentage of patients requiring long-term RRT was just 1.6% in the absence of pre-morbid renal impairment.

Coagulation

Relative hypoperfusion of tissue beds is compounded by fibrin deposition due to the imbalance between thrombogenesis and thrombolysis in sepsis. Disseminated intravascular coagulation

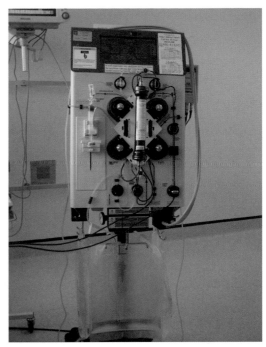

Figure 4.5 Renal replacement therapy. CVVH uses a peristaltic pump to draw venous blood from the patient and pass it through a filter, essentially a high-surface area semi-permeable membrane. Hydrostatic pressure causes water and solutes, including small and some medium-sized molecules, to pass across the filter, with the filtrate being collected in effluent bags. Isotonic replacement fluid is then added to the remaining blood before it is returned to the circulation. The extracorporeal circuit is anticoagulated using heparin, a prostaglandin or citrate to extend filter life and preserve clotting factors. CVVH is usually applied continually.

(DIC), also called consumptive coagulopathy, causes the consumption of platelets and coagulation factors and results in simultaneous thrombosis and haemorrhage. It is more commonly seen in gram-negative sepsis (particularly meningococcal sepsis) than in gram-positive sepsis. The precipitating cause is endothelial dysfunction, with resultant fibrin deposition.

There is no single test to diagnose DIC but a decreased platelet count, elevated fibrinogen degradation products (FDPs) or D-dimers, a prolonged bleeding time and decreased fibrinogen are indicators. A high index of suspicion should be maintained in the event of a disease linked to DIC (such as sepsis), single or multiple organ dysfunction and signs of ongoing consumption of coagulation products. There may be microangiopathic haemolytic anaemia (as in thrombotic thrombocytopenic purpura (TTP) and haemolytic-uremic syndrome (HUS)). The most common complications of DIC are large vessel occlusion, liver infarction, acute renal failure, coma, subarachnoid haemorrhage and multiple cortical and brainstem haemorrhages and infarction.

Central nervous system

Sepsis-associated encephalopathy (SAE) is a common complication of severe sepsis with up to 71% of patients demonstrating at least a mild degree of cerebral dysfunction. Delirium, the most common presentation of septic encephalopathy, is readily diagnosed and is independently associated with poor outcomes. The aetiology is still unknown, but a disruption of the blood–brain barrier, cerebral blood flow abnormalities and resulting cerebral cellular dysfunction have been postulated. Other processes that can contribute are listed in Box 4.1.

> **Box 4.1 Possible mechanisms for sepsis-associated encephalopathy**
>
> - Disruption of the blood–brain barrier
> - Cerebral blood flow abnormalities
> - Cerebral haemorrhage due to coagulopathy
> - Microinfarction
> - Hypoxic-ischaemic encephalopathy (HIE)
> - Metastatic cerebral abscess and/or meningitis
> - 'Cytokine storm'

The resultant delirium or confusion can be extremely difficult to manage in the ICU, as patients are uncooperative and can pose a danger to themselves. Although SAE is considered to be reversible, survivors often show a high incidence of long-term or permanent cognitive and behavioural sequelae.

Gastrointestinal

The liver appears to be fairly resistant to septic insults. Cholestatic jaundice may occur, but the gross and microscopic appearances of the liver in septic shock have no specific features. If the source of the sepsis is the biliary tract (cholangitis), abscesses may be centred on portal tracts. Hypotension may cause hepatic ischaemia; biochemically a severe rise in transaminases often occurs and there may be some peribiliary infarction.

Splanchnic hypoperfusion is a common finding that leads to increased intestinal permeability and bacterial translocation. It also contributes to upper gastrointestinal bleeding by causing stress ulceration of the gastric mucosa, which is further compounded by global coagulopathy.

Critical illness polineuropathy

Critical illness polineuropathy is a sensorimotor polineuropathy that is present in up to 70% of patients with severe sepsis. It can be difficult to diagnose due to the severe sepsis, use of neuromuscular blocking agents to facilitate ventilation and presence of encephalopathy. The condition usually only becomes apparent when difficulties are encountered on weaning the patient from mechanical ventilation. The findings are a flaccid weakness of extremities with absent deep tendon reflexes. The cause is a degeneration of sensory and motor axons. The prognosis is related to the severity of the disease and the age of the patient. Muscle weakness is common at 2 months after discharge from intensive therapy unit (ITU) and can still be demonstrated up to 6 months later.

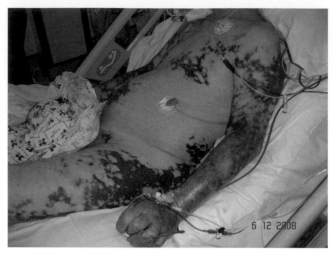

Figure 4.6 Purpura fulminans.

Immunological

Although severe sepsis is an acute, deadly disease, survivors of the acute episode carry a 1-year mortality of up to 26%, mostly due to pulmonary complications. In fact, the risk of dying is higher than the general population for up to 8 years after the septic episode. The underlying reason seems to be a dysregulation of the immune response and a degree of immunosuppression, possibly mediated by chemokines and cytokines.

Skin and limbs

Purpura fulminans (Figure 4.6) is a haemorrhagic condition characterized by cutaneous haemorrhage and necrosis, usually in the presence of DIC. Histologically, there are microvascular thrombi in the dermis which result in perivascular haemorrhage and necrosis but with minimal inflammation. Purpura fulminans is most commonly associated with *Neisseria meningitidis* and pneumococcal septicaemia but can be seen in any blood-borne infection with encapsulated organisms. As the blisters and necrotic skin begin to organize and resolve, they may become infected and be a further source of sepsis. Large deficits may leave unsightly scarring and may need surgical debridement.

In addition, severe sepsis may be associated with vasoconstriction severe enough to cause infarction of digits and even distal limbs (in children). Poorly fluid-resuscitated patients treated with vasoconstrictors alone can develop skin and limb infarction and auto-amputation.

Psychological

The prolonged duration of stay in the ICU has been associated with an increased incidence of depression and anxiety. Up to 20% of ARDS patients meet diagnostic criteria for post-traumatic stress disorder (PTSD). Panic attacks are common, even at night, and

40% of sufferers require long-term treatment. Social isolation, a dependence on others and a fear of being alone or in crowded places occur frequently. Health-related quality of life (HRQL) can show a marked reduction for up to 2 years after hospitalization, with common complaints being greater depression and dependence, physical symptoms and reduced sexual activity.

Conclusion

Severe sepsis is a fulminant disease process that can rapidly cause significant dysfunction in most of the body systems, in most cases resulting in life-threatening loss of homeostasis. The fact that sepsis can lead to failure of the cardiovascular, respiratory and renal system at the same time makes it especially dangerous with high mortality rates despite organ replacement and support. The complication rates from most of the supportive therapies further compound the problem. Vast amounts of resources are spent yearly on managing these patients in ICUs, where despite our best efforts, they can be exposed to multi-drug-resistant pathogens.

Further reading

Ely EW & Goyette RE. Sepsis with acute organ dysfunction. In: Hall JB, Schmidt GA & Wood LDH, eds. *Principles of Critical Care*. McGraw-Hill, USA, 2005: 699–733.

Kutsogiannis NT. Quality of Life after intensive care. In: Ridley S, ed. *Outcomes in Critical Care*. Butterworth-Heinemann, 2002: 139–168.

Ware LB & Matthay MA. The acute respiratory distress syndrome. *New England Journal of Medicine* 2000; **342** (18): 1334–1349.

CHAPTER 5

The Pathophysiology of Sepsis

Edwin Mitchell[1] and Tony Whitehouse[2]

[1]West Midlands Deanery, Birmingham, UK
[2]University Hospitals Birmingham, Birmingham, UK

OVERVIEW

- Sepsis is a systemic disease, probably triggered by overactivation of the innate immune system

- Multiple pathways combine synergistically to produce the clinical picture

- Organ dysfunction secondary to systemic inflammation characterizes sepsis

- Cardiovascular changes are most profound. Absolute anuria and acute renal failure (ARF) are common but if the patient recovers, organ function is likely to revert back to pre-morbid states.

"Our arsenals for fighting off bacteria are so powerful, and involve so many different mechanisms, that we are in more danger from them than from the invaders. We live in the midst of explosive devices . . . " Lewis Thomas (1972).

It is more than 35 years since the article containing this quotation was published. In that time, the mortality rate from sepsis has fallen from an estimated 60% to approximately 30%. This improvement is almost entirely due to earlier recognition of the critically ill patient, better intensive care facilities and more effective use of existing therapies rather than due to any marked translation of laboratory research into new and useful clinical treatments. There have been advances in the understanding of the mechanisms and pathophysiology of sepsis; it is now clear that multiple pathways are involved in the development of sepsis, and it is probably insufficient to treat any one of them in isolation (Figure 5.1, Table 5.1).

Pro-inflammatory responses to infection

Sepsis is a collection of physiological responses to an infectious agent. Clinical signs such as fever, tachycardia and hypotension are common, but the clinical course depends on the type of infectious organism, the site and size of the infecting insult and

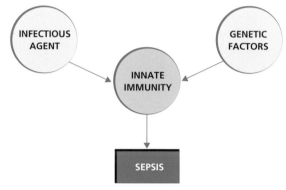

Figure 5.1 Interaction between host and agent in the development of sepsis.

the genetically determined properties of the host's immune system (Figure 5.2).

Examples:
- Organisms such as *Neisseria meningitidis* seem to provoke a rapidly progressive illness with severe cardiovascular collapse. On the other hand some organisms (certain fungi) have a more subtle presentation.
- The sudden introduction of large numbers of bacteria into sterile areas of the body, such as bowel rupture, may also prompt severe illness whereas subcutaneous infection may be contained for longer.

Table 5.1 Some of the treatments tried unsuccessfully in the management of sepsis.

Methylprednisolone
Hyperimmune immunoglobulin
Endotoxin antibody
Bactericidal permeability increasing protein
Tumour necrosis factor antibody
Soluble tumour necrosis factor receptor antibody
Interleukin 1 receptor antagonist
Platelet-activating factor antagonists
Bradykinin antagonists
Ibuprofen
Antithrombin III
N-acetyl cysteine
Procysteine
Nitric oxide synthase inhibitor (L-monomethyl NG-arginine (L-NMMA))

ABC of Sepsis. Edited by Ron Daniels and Tim Nutbeam. © 2010 by Blackwell Publishing, ISBN: 978-1-4501-8194-5.

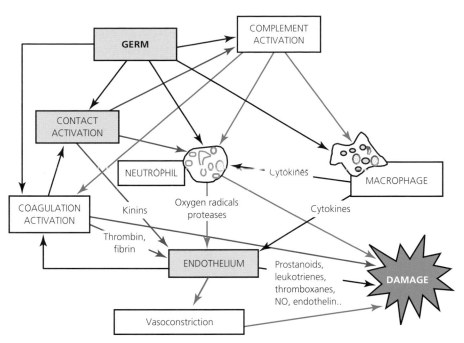

Figure 5.2 Some of the multiple pathways involved in the development of sepsis. NO, nitric oxide. Courtesy: Prof. Mervyn Singer.

- Genetic polymorphisms of toll-like receptor 4 (TLR-4) are associated with a predisposition to shock with gram-negative organisms, and mutations in the tumour necrosis factor α (TNF-α) receptor affect outcomes from severe sepsis.

The innate (non-specific) immune system

The innate immune system, comprising cellular (polymorphonuclear leukocytes, macrophages, natural killer cells, dendritic cells) and humoral components (complement and coagulation systems), is activated in early sepsis. Its role is to limit bacterial growth and replication, and ultimately to remove organisms (Table 5.2). The response of the innate immune response is complex, with multiple, complementary systems each with amplification steps.

Cellular response to infection

Activation via toll-like receptors (TLRs)

Perhaps the most studied pathway by which bacterial sepsis is initiated is through the outer cell products of gram-negative and gram-positive bacteria binding to TLRs. To do this, they often use an intermediary binding molecule such as CD14 (Figure 5.3). At least 10 TLRs have been described in humans; all are transmembrane proteins with an intracellular domain that binds protein kinases when activated. They are widely found on leukocytes and macrophages, and some types on endothelial cells. Different TLRs have specificity for different bacterial, fungal or viral products. The specificities of some TLRs are given in Table 5.3.

Activation of the innate immune system results in liberation of reactive oxygen species, nitric oxide (NO), proteases and

Table 5.2 Interactions between the innate immune system and pathogens.

Pathogen	Main examples	Cell phagocytosis?	Complement
Viruses	*Rhinovirus*, influenza, measles, mumps	Natural killer cells	No
Intracellular bacteria	*Mycobacteria, Listeria monocytogenes, Legionella*	Neutrophils and natural killer cells	No
	Rickettsia	No	No
Extracellular bacteria	*Staphylococcus, Streptococcus, Neisseria, Salmonella typhii*	Neutrophils	Yes
Intracellular protozoa	*Plasmodium malariae, Leishmaniasis*	No	No
Extracellular protozoa	*Giardia lamblia, Entamoeba histolytica*	Macrophage	Yes
Extracellular fungi	*Candida, Cryptococcus*	No	Yes

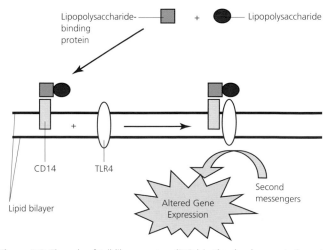

Figure 5.3 The role of toll-like receptors (TLRs) in the development of sepsis.

Table 5.3 Specificities of toll-like receptors.

Toll-like receptor number	Specificity
1	Lipopeptides, lipoteichoic acid
2	Peptidoglycan
3	Double-stranded RNA (viral)
4	Lipopolysaccharide
5	Bacterial flagella
6	Lipopeptides, lipoteichoic acid
9	Microbial DNA

pore-forming molecules, bringing about bacterial killing. Some of these molecules also directly damage the patient's own cells and may cause tissue dysfunction by other means; for example, NO inactivates circulating catecholamines (epinephrine and norepinephrine) and has been implicated in sepsis-induced mitochondrial dysfunction (see below).

The innate immune system also causes release of inflammatory cytokines such as TNF-α and interleukins 1 and 6. These further prime and activate nearby immune cells. Disappointingly, blocking the action of individual early inflammatory cytokines has not improved clinical outcomes in established human sepsis (Table 5.1), despite early promising work in animal models.

Vascular endothelium

The vascular endothelium plays a major role in the host's defence to an invading organism but also in the development of sepsis. Activated endothelium not only allows the adhesion and migration of stimulated immune cells but also becomes porous to large molecules, resulting in tissue oedema.

Evidence is emerging that the endothelium is also selective in its actions. For example, control of white cell movement is predominantly located in post-capillary venules, whereas regulation of vasomotor tone is mainly arteriolar. Stimulated endothelial cells produce NO that causes, amongst other actions, vascular smooth muscle relaxation. Vasodilatation opens up collateral channels through tissues, reducing both perfusion pressure and blood flow through capillary networks.

Mitochondria and tissue perfusion

It is open to discussion whether microvascular dysfunction and disruption of blood flow or disruption of mitochondrial energy pathways are more important to the development of organ failure.

A combination of shunting of blood through collateral channels, physical obstruction from microthrombi and an increase in blood viscosity from loss of red cell flexibility results in disordered blood flow through capillary beds. Patients with sepsis have been shown to have a reduced number of perfused capillaries, sluggish flow in those capillaries still open, and capillary oedema that further reduces their diameter (Figure 5.4). Oxygen and other nutrients thus have further to diffuse from capillary to cell. Organs may then become hypoxic even though gross blood flow to an organ may increase.

In addition to shunting impairing oxygen supply to some capillary beds, NO has direct effects on the mitochondrial oxygen transport chain. By combining with oxygen free radicals (O_2^-), NO can go on to produce peroxynitrite ($ONOO^-$). All three compounds are potent free radicals that combine either reversibly or irreversibly with proteins of the electron transport chain (including succinate dehydrogenase and cytochrome c oxidase).

Through either mechanism, cellular energy levels (as measured by adenosine triphosphate (ATP)) fall as metabolic activity begins to exceed production. It is possible that cellular dysfunction (and even cell death) derives from falling intra-cellular ATP concentrations. This could explain why relatively few histological changes are found at autopsy and the eventual resolution of severe symptoms such as complete anuria and hypotension.

Humoral response to sepsis

Activation of the complement cascade occurs via non-specific interactions with bacterial or viral cell surfaces, or via binding antibodies and proteins such as mannose binding lectin that are attached to the infectious organism. The activated complement cascade releases many fragments, such as C3b and C5a, that powerfully attract leukocytes and perpetuate the immune response.

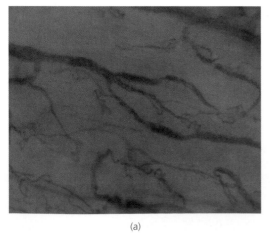 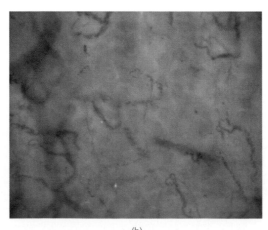

(a)   (b)

Figure 5.4 Orthogonal polarization spectral image of the microcirculation during sepsis (b) and in health (a). Courtesy: Prof. C Ince and Dr P Goedhart, Amsterdam, Holland.

Compensatory Anti-inflammatory Reaction Syndrome (CARS)

Patients during the later (>72 hours) and recovery phases of sepsis frequently acquire new infections, often with bacteria and fungi usually thought to be of low pathogenic potential. These patients may not exhibit the overwhelming vascular responses seen in 'new' episodes of sepsis. Relative immunosuppression may derive from a change in the balance of pro-inflammatory and anti-inflammatory cytokines (Figure 5.5), catecholamine-induced immunosuppression and an alteration in the T helper cell responses. Studies on T lymphocytes of patients with sepsis have shown that they are in a state of non-responsiveness (*anergy*, sometimes referred to as

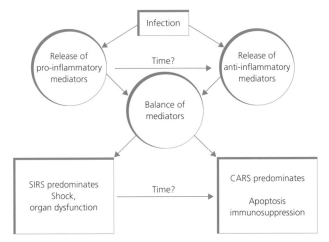

Figure 5.5 Pro-inflammatory and anti-inflammatory mediators are released in response to infection (although this is somewhat an artificial distinction as some molecules may exhibit both pro-inflammatory and anti-inflammatory actions). The balance between pro- and anti-inflammatory mediators may dictate the clinical course of the patient.

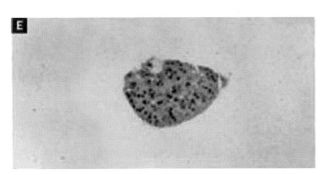

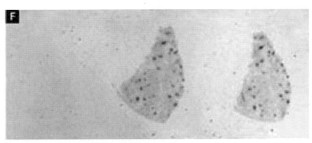

Figure 5.6 Unmagnified view of two microscope slides of spleens from patients with trauma (panel E) and patients who died of sepsis (panel F), with staining for B cells (CD20). Taken from Hotchkiss R & Karl I. The pathophysiology and treatment of sepsis. *New England Journal of Medicine* 2003; **348**: 138–150 with permission.

leukocyte reprogramming) and that apoptosis (programmed cell death) is occurring amongst B lymphocytes in the spleen. (Figure 5.6).

Organ-specific pathophysiology

The circulatory system in sepsis

Vascular smooth muscle has a reduced sensitivity to catecholamines in sepsis, and large amounts of exogenous catecholamines may be required to reverse the extreme vasodilatation seen. This may be due to a combination of reduced catecholamine receptor density on affected cells, abnormal potassium channel responsiveness and deactivation of catecholamines by NO. Relative deficiencies of vasopressin from the pituitary and corticosteroids from the adrenal glands have been noted in some of the patients with severe sepsis. The mechanisms for these observations are unclear but there is evidence to suggest that the brain, through a hypothalamic-pituitary-adrenal axis, may have a role. Exogenous steroids and vasopressin may restore catecholamine responsiveness, but are not proven to affect mortality.

The heart in sepsis

The heart may be severely affected in sepsis. Patients are typically tachycardic, and markers of myocardial injury such as troponins I and T can appear in the blood, even in the absence of coronary artery disease. Although myocardial hypoperfusion has been proposed as a mechanism, coronary blood flow in patients with sepsis was shown to be elevated in one study. No difference in blood flow was found between patients who developed myocardial dysfunction and those who did not. Furthermore, the heart's consumption of oxygen and production of lactate and high-energy phosphates are preserved in septic shock, suggesting that heart dysfunction in these patients is not related to perfusion.

As far back as the 1980s, researchers combined serum from patients with sepsis with healthy myocytes and noted a correlation between the degree of *in vivo* cardiac depression and reduction in myocyte contractility. However, no substance has been identified as responsible for this effect.

The marked drop in systemic vascular resistance results in a reduction in left ventricular afterload and an increase in cardiac output in the early phases of sepsis, but to sustain this demands higher left atrial filling pressures and a greater end-diastolic volume than would normally occur in health. This is represented as an upward shift of the Starling curve and is suggestive of myocardial dysfunction. The left ventricle may dilate acutely, a change that reverts to normal in survivors 7–10 days after the onset of sepsis. Interestingly, this seems to be an adaptive response as non-survivors do not exhibit ventricular dilatation. The right heart also dilates and contracts less efficiently in patients with sepsis. Although pulmonary vascular resistance is often raised, this by itself is not sufficient to explain a reduced right ventricular ejection fraction, again suggesting direct myocardial depression.

Myocardial depression, and the failure to maintain elevated filling pressures, is implicated in the decompensation seen in later phases of sepsis when the circulation changes from hyperdynamic (with warm, well-perfused peripheries) to hypodynamic (with peripheral circulatory collapse). Put another way, shock becomes a combination of hypovolaemia (relative due to vasodilatation and absolute due to fluid shifts) and cardiac insufficiency.

The lung in sepsis

The lung is involved early in the inflammatory process, with endothelial leakage of fluids and proteins into the interstitium, infiltration of activated neutrophils, and loss of surfactant. Later, mononuclear cells infiltrate, type II pneumocytes proliferate and interstitial fibrosis may develop. Inflammatory pulmonary oedema (defined by the absence of raised left atrial pressure) may develop, manifesting clinically as acute lung injury or acute respiratory distress syndrome (ARDS) (Figure 5.7).

Mechanical ventilation is frequently necessary in these patients and may worsen the tissue damage by further inducing release of pro-inflammatory cytokines. Protective ventilation with lower tidal volumes and higher positive end-expiratory pressure (PEEP) has been shown to reduce cytokine production and improve patient survival.

The kidney in sepsis

Acute renal failure (ARF) induced by sepsis remains an enigma. Unexplained features include the *absence* of significant histological change, despite anuria and biochemical derangement and the *lag time for recovery* of renal function that may take up to several months despite early resolution of systemic inflammation and restoration of a normal circulatory profile. Most intensive care unit (ICU) patients diagnosed with sepsis become independent of renal replacement therapy and patients with normal renal function before their septic episode revert to having normal creatinine levels with time.

Although the term *acute tubular necrosis* (ATN) is colloquially applied to the renal dysfunction of sepsis, histology fails to reveal either necrosis or overt signs of tubular damage. NO may again be implicated in sepsis-induced renal dysfunction. Not only is NO responsible for the distribution of blood between renal cortex and medulla but tubular function is also highly energy dependent (as stated before, NO has direct and indirect effects on mitochondrial energy production). There is also activation of the renin–angiotensin–aldosterone system. Hypotension results in increased sympathetic tone and the release of vasopressin from

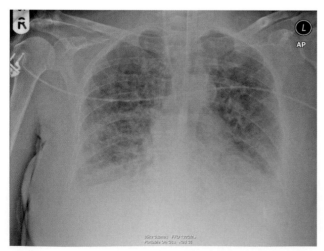

Figure 5.7 Chest radiograph of acute respiratory distress syndrome.

Table 5.4 Clinical signs in sepsis and their cause and mechanisms.

Sign	Cause	Mechanism
Hypotension	Vasodilatation	Nitric oxide
		Interleukin 1
		Bradykinin
		Histamine
		PAF
		Catecholamine resistance
	Relative hypovolaemia	Vasodilatation
		Capillary leakage
	Myocardial depression	Unknown factors
Hypoxaemia	Hyperventilation	Acidosis
		Shunt and V/Q mismatch
		Pulmonary infiltration and oedema
	Increased metabolic demand	Redistribution of blood flow
Oliguria	Reduced glomerular filtration rate	Relative hypovolaemia
		Hypotension
		Low cardiac output
		Endothelin
		Microthrombi
	Impaired tubular function	Nitric oxide
		Renin–angiotensin–aldosterone system
Confusion	Disruption of intra-cerebral blood flow	Possible build-up of cerebral 'toxins'
		Direct neural synapse disruption
		Hypotension
		Low cardiac output
		Microthrombi
Failure to absorb from GI tract		Hypotension
		Possible direct effect
Liver failure	Disruption of blood flow	Hypotension
		Diversion of blood flow
		Low cardiac output
		Microthrombi

PAF, platelet-activating factor; GI, gastrointestinal.

the pituitary. The resulting vasoconstriction causes sodium and water retention and a predisposition to ARF. Endothelin, another pressor hormone, is elevated in sepsis, and in combination with neutrophil adhesion and microthrombi, reduces glomerular blood flow and filtration.

A summary of the clinical signs seen in severe sepsis, with the physiological process responsible and the means by which this dysfunction is produced ('effector', where known) is given in Table 5.4.

Acknowledgements

The authors wish to thank Prof. M Singer, London and Prof. C Ince and Dr P Goedhart, Amsterdam for allowing publication of Figures 5.1 and 5.4.

Further reading

Abraham E & Singer M. Mechanisms of sepsis-induced organ dysfunction. *Critical Care Medicine* 2007; **35** (10): 2408–2416. Review PMID: 17948334

Remick D. Pathophysiology of sepsis. *American Journal of Pathology* 2007; **170** (5): 1435–1444. Review.

Thomas L. Germs. *New England Journal of Medicine* 1972; **287**: 553–555.

CHAPTER 6

Initial Resuscitation

Tim Nutbeam

West Midlands School of Emergency Medicine, University Hospitals Birmingham, Birmingham, UK

OVERVIEW

- Initial assessment and resuscitation of the patient with sepsis should follow the ABCDE format
- Resuscitation is time critical in sepsis. Unnecessary delays will impact adversely on outcome
- Oxygen delivery to the tissues must be optimized to meet increased demand
- Accurate monitoring will indicate the need for, and response to, targeted resuscitation
- Immediate therapy and diagnostic support should be undertaken concurrently, with the likely source of sepsis identified and contained early

---

As we have ascertained in previous chapters, patients with sepsis are critically ill and need to be treated in an efficient and effective manner. Sepsis is a time-critical disease process – prompt aggressive initial resuscitation unequivocally reduces long-term morbidity and mortality.

Initial resuscitation consists of a number of simple steps of care, each of which is well within the remit of the most junior members of the nursing/medical team. However, patients with sepsis should always be assessed by senior medical staff at the earliest opportunity, with early involvement of the critical care team if organ dysfunction is present.

Patients should be assessed and resuscitated using the ABCDE approach (Box 6.1).

Box 6.1 **The ABCDE approach**

A = Airway assessment, maintenance and oxygen
B = Breathing and ventilation assessment
C = Circulation assessment, intravenous (IV) access and fluids
D = Disability: assess the neurological status and check the blood glucose
E = Exposure and environmental control

ABC of Sepsis. Edited by Ron Daniels and Tim Nutbeam. © 2010 by Blackwell Publishing, ISBN: 978-1-4501-8194-5.

By assessing the patient in this methodical manner immediately, life-threatening pathology should be identified and treated – remember sepsis may not be the sole pathology.

The ABCDE approach is covered in detail in courses such as Advanced Life Support (ALS), Acute Life-Threatening Events Recognition and Treatment (ALERT) and Survive Sepsis.

The goal of initial resuscitation is to return the patient's physiological parameters to within normal limits. The resuscitation phase consists of three processes:

- optimizing oxygen delivery and tissue perfusion;
- careful monitoring of vital signs and end organ function to guide further resuscitation;
- instituting strategies aimed at containing or removing the source of infection.

These processes are designed to stop (or at least slow down) the onset of the multi-organ dysfunction syndrome responsible for the extremely high mortality in severe sepsis.

Once sepsis has been identified, and a thorough ABCDE assessment performed, the following steps should all be achieved as soon as possible. Some of these therapies – high-flow oxygen, cannulation, fluid challenges, urinary output monitoring – may already be in progress as a result of the global resuscitation strategy; if they are not, they should be undertaken immediately. The steps below provide a logical order in which to provide treatment: the aim is to complete all of the steps within 1 hour. The approach to resuscitation in severe sepsis is summarized in Box 6.2.

Box 6.2 **Summary of approach to resuscitation in severe sepsis**

1. Perform ABCDE assessment, initiate immediate therapy
   May include: Clinical assessment
   Airway support
   High-flow oxygen
   Cannulation
   Fluid challenges
   Urine output monitoring
   Blood glucose measurement
   Temperature regulation

2. Cross check to ensure that the following have been performed:
   High-flow oxygen therapy
   Cannulation

Fluid challenges if circulation compromised
Urine output monitoring

3. Perform diagnostics specific to sepsis:
    May include: Cultures (blood and others)
                  Lactate measurement
                  Haemoglobin and other blood tests
                  Imaging to identify source

4. Complete therapies specific to sepsis:
                  IV broad-spectrum antibiotics
                  Surgical or percutaneous drainage if possible

As an *aide-memoire*, a subset of these tasks has been described as
the 'Sepsis Six' (www.survivesepsis.org):
                  High-flow oxygen
                  Blood cultures (and others)
                  IV broad-spectrum antibiotics
                  IV fluid challenges
                  Measure haemoglobin and lactate
                  Monitor accurate urine output

High-flow oxygen

Sepsis dramatically increases the body's metabolic rate and thereby its oxygen requirements. In order to maximize the amount of oxygen available for respiration, patients should be given high-flow oxygen via a non-rebreathe face mask with reservoir bag. Patients should have their haemoglobin oxygen saturation measured by a pulse oximeter – saturation should be kept at $\geq 94\%$ unless they have documented chronic hypoxaemia (Figure 6.1).

Recent British Thoracic Society guidelines for the administration of oxygen advise the use of the lowest possible concentration of inspired oxygen to achieve a target saturation. However, the guidelines acknowledge that this is inappropriate in the critically ill including patients with sepsis, and in these circumstances advocate the use of high-flow oxygen.

The non-rebreathe mask is not suitable for long-term oxygen therapy, but is essential for the acute resuscitation phase to maximize arterial oxygen content. If the patient's haemoglobin oxygen saturation is below 94% or the patient is worsening (increasing respiratory rate, poor respiratory effort, decreasing level of consciousness) senior medical or Critical Care assistance should be immediately requested.

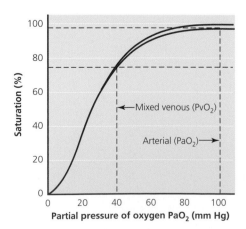

Figure 6.1 Graph saturations against PaO_2.

Chronic obstructive pulmonary disease (COPD) patients with type II respiratory failure may not respond well to high-flow oxygen. A proportion of these patients rely on what is referred to as a 'hypoxic drive' – if the oxygen content of their blood rises above a certain level, they may lose their respiratory stimulus. These patients need to be intensively monitored and have regular arterial blood gases (ABGs) performed. These patients will undoubtedly require some supplemental oxygen, though this may be most appropriately delivered through a venturi (fixed performance, high flow) system. Early senior medical review is essential.

Cannulation

It is imperative to acquire and maintain good IV access. At least one (more may be required) large-bore cannula should be placed in a peripheral vein using an aseptic no-touch technique. The largest cannula possible according to the clinician's level of expertise and the individual patient's veins should be inserted. The larger the radius of the cannula, the quicker fluid challenges may be given (Table 6.1).

Blood cultures

These should be acquired before (but should not delay) the administration of IV antibiotics. Blood cultures should be taken percutaneously and before flushing newly placed IV access devices. They should also be taken from every indwelling catheter or cannula, and appropriate cultures should also be considered from other sources (Table 6.2). Blood cultures will not affect the choice of initial broad-spectrum antibiotic but will aid in future antibiotic choices once the pathogen has been identified.

It is important to place an adequate sample (normally 10 ml of blood) in each bottle, using a recommended aseptic technique. This

Table 6.1 Cannula sizes, flow rates, colours and uses.

Colour	Size	Flow rate		Use
Blue	22G	36 ml/min	2.2 l/h	Paediatric or elderly patients with small, fragile veins
Pink	20G	61 ml/min	3.7 l/h	IV maintenance fluids, drugs, blood products
Green	18G	90 ml/min	5.4 l/h	
White	17G	140 ml/min	6.2 l/h	Rapid infusions of fluids, drugs and blood products.
Grey	16G	200 ml/min	12 l/h	Unstable patients, emergency situations
Brown/orange	14G	300 ml/min	18 l/h	

Table 6.2 Examples of sources of sepsis, cultures to take and potential pathogens.

Source	Sample	Potential pathogen
Urinary tract	Urine	*Escherichia coli, Proteus, Klebsiella*
Meningitis	Cerebrospinal fluid	*Streptococcus pneumoniae, Neisseria meningitidis, Haemophilus influenzae, E. coli*
Cellulitis	Skin swab	*Group A Streptococcus, Staphylococcus*
Epiglottitis	Epiglottic swab	*H. influenzae type B, S. pneumoniae*
Lungs	Sputum	*S. pneumoniae, Staphylococcus aureus, H. influenzae, Klebsiella pneumoniae, E. coli*

increases the culture's sensitivity whilst reducing the risk of sample contamination. Blood culture sampling technique is covered in detail in the next chapter.

Other blood tests

A full blood screen at this point will aid in the identification of organ dysfunction and give a baseline to compare future tests. This may consist of urea and electrolytes, liver function tests, full blood count and a clotting profile.

It is recommended that if a patient's haemoglobin has dropped below 7 g/dl that an urgent cross-match sample be taken and the patient be transfused with packed red cells to above this level. As haemoglobin is essential for the transport of oxygen around the body, it is vital to optimize haemoglobin levels to reduce organ dysfunction. Studies evaluating the effectiveness of early goal-directed therapy (EGDT) in sepsis have demonstrated improved outcomes with transfusion to a haemoglobin concentration of >10 g/dl, although this higher target is not universally accepted.

Lactate measurement

Lactate can be measured from a venous sample sent urgently to the biochemistry laboratory or using an ABG syringe and an appropriately calibrated blood gas analyser.

Lactate accumulates as a result of anaerobic respiration – the more anaerobic respiration that occurs, the higher the lactate. Lactate gives us an indication of prognosis (Figure 6.2), acts as a guide for fluid administration and enables the clinician to judge progress within the initial resuscitation phase. In patients with severe sepsis and a normal blood pressure, elevated lactate levels were demonstrated in 25% in one study. These patients are described as having 'cryptic shock'.

Procalcitonin is an appropriate alternative to lactate measurement in identifying the extent of hypoperfusion. It may be more specific to the septic process than lactate, but is not widely available currently.

Fluid challenges

Judicious early fluid challenges are key to the management of sepsis. Much controversy exists over whether a colloid (for example, Voluven®) or a crystalloid (for example, Hartmann's solution, 0.9% saline) is more appropriate in the acute resuscitative phase. Large meta-analysis of the various clinical trials has yet supplied no conclusive answer to this quandary. Associations of renal dysfunction with starch-containing colloids and hyperchloraemic metabolic acidosis with large volumes of 0.9% saline currently lead many to favour Hartmann's solution and gelatin-based colloids.

If patients with sepsis are hypotensive or if they show other signs of circulatory insufficiency (for example, high serum lactate), fluid challenges of 10 ml/kg of colloid or 20 ml/kg of crystalloid should be administered in divided boluses with reassessment of physiological parameters between each bolus. This fluid challenge can be repeated twice, up to a total of three boluses (equivalent of 60 ml/kg of crystalloid). This can represent nearly 5 litres of IV fluid being delivered appropriately and safely within the early phases of resuscitation in an average person. Caution should be exhibited in those patients known to have heart failure. However, on acute presentation, even this group of patients usually have a depleted intravascular volume (they are 'dry') and will require some judicious fluid resuscitation.

If a patient remains hypotensive following fluid challenges (or is known to have heart failure) a central venous catheter (CVC) should be inserted by a clinician trained in this procedure. The CVC will allow the monitoring of central venous pressure as well as the administration of vasopressors and inotropes when necessary.

Intravenous broad-spectrum antibiotics

The evidence shows that early administration of appropriate broad-spectrum IV antibiotics has a major effect on mortality from sepsis (Figure 6.3).

It is therefore key not only to prescribe the appropriate antibiotics but also to ensure that they are administered in a timely fashion. Appropriate choice of broad-spectrum agent will take into account the following:

- any allergies the patient is known to have;
- the patient's clinical condition and likely source of infection;
- local policies related to antibiotic administration;
- previous antibiotic administration.

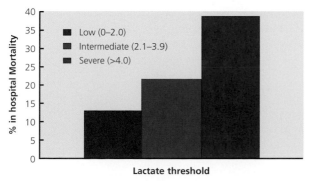

Figure 6.2 Graph of mortality against lactate, n = 1613. From Trzeciak S et al. 2007.

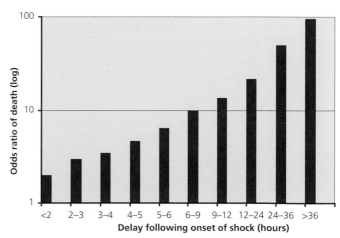

Figure 6.3 Mortality increases with delay in antibiotics following onset of septic shock. From Kumar A et al. 2006.

Potential sites, likely pathogens and examples of appropriate broad-spectrum antibiotics can be found in the next chapter.

If a patient is known or suspected to be neutropenic or immuno-compromised, it is essential to urgently discuss the case with a senior haematologist and microbiologist (see Chapter 12 for more details).

Accurate monitoring of urine output

In normal circumstances the body's autoregulatory system ensures that renal blood flow stays within normal limits across a wide range of blood pressures (Figure 6.4). In sepsis this function is disabled to a certain extent: if a patient's blood pressure is low, renal blood flow will be low; consequentially there will be a fall in urine output.

A urinary catheter allows the accurate measurement of urine output from the kidneys, giving a direct estimation of renal blood flow. This enables the clinician to judge renal perfusion and is an early predictor of renal failure.

Should the patient remain fully mobile and cooperative, then it may be appropriate to avoid additional risks posed by catheterization and allow self-voiding. The key, however, remains the accurate hourly measurement of hourly output and in practice this will be appropriate in only a few patients.

The clinician should aim for a normal physiological urine output. A patient is defined as oliguric if the urine output is <0.5 ml/kg/hour over 2 successive hours. Persistent oliguria is a sign of impending renal failure. Anuria (very low or no urine output) may indicate that the kidneys have completely failed, but more commonly represents a blocked or kinked catheter and this should be excluded.

Endpoint

The endpoint for the initial resuscitation phase will come when all the above steps have been completed. At this stage, either:

- the initial resuscitation has been successful and the patient's physiology will have normalized;

- the resuscitation alone has not been successful; more advanced resuscitative measures using invasive monitoring and vasoactive drugs will be required.

Suggested goals for resuscitation endpoints are as follows:

- Mean arterial blood pressure >65 mmHg
- Improving capillary refill time
- Warming of extremities
- Urine output >0.5 ml/kg/hour
- Improving mental status
- Decreasing lactate

Successful resuscitation

At this stage, the patients still have the potential to become critically ill. They should be nursed in an acute ward where regular (at least hourly) observations should be taken. If they deteriorate they should be promptly assessed by senior medical personnel. It is important that the patient continues on appropriate first-line antibiotics until the course is finished, or is advised otherwise by the microbiologist. All cultures taken should be followed up and appropriate action taken. In certain infections, the public health authority should be informed and contact tracing carried out.

Unsuccessful initial resuscitation

An urgent referral should be made to senior medical/intensive care personnel. A central line should be inserted by an appropriately trained individual and if required vasopressors and/or inotropes commenced. If a patient has respiratory failure he or she may require intubation and positive pressure ventilation. Appropriate additional organ support, for example, renal replacement therapy should be started at the earliest opportunity. The patient will require nursing in a high dependency area. These issues are covered in detail in subsequent chapters.

Further reading

Daniels R, Nutbeam T & Laver K. Survive Sepsis manual. *The Official Training Programme of the Surviving Sepsis Campaign*, 1st edn, 2007.

Dellinger RP, Levy MM & Carlet JM. Surviving Sepsis Campaign: international guidelines for the management of severe sepsis and septic shock: 2008. *Intensive Care Medicine* 2008; **34**: 17–60.

Kumar A, Roberts D, Wood K *et al.* Duration of hypotension before initiation of effective antimicrobial therapy is the determinant of survival in human septic shock. *Critical Care Medicine* 2006; **34** (6): 1589–1596.

Rivers E, Nguyen B, Havstad S *et al.* Early goal directed therapy in the treatment of severe sepsis and septic shock. *New England Journal of Medicine* 2001; **345**: 1368–1377.

Trzeciak F, Dellinger R, Chansky M *et al.* Serum lactate as a predictor of mortality in patients with infection. *Academic Emergency Medicine* 2007; **13**: 1150–1151.

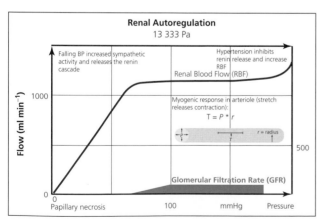

Figure 6.4 Graph of blood pressure and urine output with and without sepsis. Blue line = without sepsis. Purple line = with sepsis.

CHAPTER 7

Microbiology and Antibiotic Therapy

Partha De[1] and Ron Daniels[2]

[1]Consultant Microbiologist, Good Hope Hospital, Birmingham, UK
[2]Good Hope Hospital, Heart of England NHS Foundation Trust, Birmingham, UK

OVERVIEW

- Infection prevention and control measures must be adhered to
- Sepsis is usually bacterial in origin, though fungi and viruses should also be considered
- General advice cannot replace in-depth knowledge of the local prevalence of pathogens and their resistance profiles
- Obtaining appropriate microbiology samples will facilitate a change from broad-spectrum to narrow-spectrum antibiotics within 48–72 hours
- The choice of antibiotic should be carefully considered

Introduction

The microbiology behind sepsis is varied, although certain organisms give rise to sepsis more commonly than others. The majority of cases encountered in the hospital setting will be bacterial, although fungal sepsis is increasing in frequency (Box 7.1).

Box 7.1 **Frequent microbial causes of sepsis**

Common
Streptococcus pneumoniae
Escherichia coli
Streptococcus pyogenes (beta-haemolytic group A)
Staphylococcus aureus including methicillin-resistant *Staphylococcus aureus* (MRSA)
Less common
Klebsiella spp and other coliforms/extended spectrum beta-lactamase (ESBL) producing organisms
Beta-haemolytic streptococci groups C and G
Candida albicans
Anaerobes (*Bacteroides fragilis*, *Clostridium* spp)

A commitment to the prevention of infection is essential to control the impact of this condition. This is covered fully in the next chapter, but its importance cannot be overstated. Infection control practices must be embraced at personal, organizational and national levels.

Good infection control practice can reduce the risk of cross infection, which in in-patients may be with pathogenic organisms resistant to multiple antibiotics. The creation of a culture in which invasive devices are inserted and handled only when necessary and with appropriate aseptic precautions, and in which prophylactic antibiotics are used judiciously, can reduce the risk of infection. Care bundles are available, for example, to prevent ventilator-associated pneumonia, and to insert and care for peripheral venous cannulae.

When used in the treatment of any infection, and particularly in those giving rise to sepsis and severe sepsis, antibiotics should target the most likely organisms (an example of a microbiology guideline is given in Figure 7.1). The choice of antibiotic (or antifungal agent) is determined by the body site of infection, by the distinction between hospital- and community-acquired infections, by the possibility of resistant organisms and by local flora and bacterial ecology. Empirical antibiotics should be started when no obvious site can be identified and subsequently rationalized (the spectrum 'narrowed') if cultures identify a pathogen. Whichever antibiotic is chosen, it should be administered promptly as delay leads to an increase in mortality.

It must be remembered that whilst antibiotics alone are effective in uncomplicated infections such as cystitis, the therapy of sepsis does not rely solely on antibiotics. The presence of systemic inflammation and organ dysfunction demands physiological assessment and often organ support. Collections of pus – for example, intra-abdominal abscesses – are unlikely to respond to antibiotics alone and will require drainage. Necrotic tissue must be excised, and infected prostheses and indwelling devices should be removed. Necrotizing fasciitis is an excellent example. This condition is a surgical emergency. Antibiotics are secondary in urgency to the surgeon's scalpel, and delay in diagnosis or inappropriate management using antibiotics alone is likely to be fatal. Before any therapy can begin, the diagnosis of sepsis must be considered, established and the cause (organism and source) identified.

Microbiological sampling in sepsis

Samples from patients must always be taken, but sampling must not cause a delay in the management of the patient and initiation

ABC of Sepsis. Edited by Ron Daniels and Tim Nutbeam. © 2010 by Blackwell Publishing, ISBN: 978-1-4501-8194-5.

First-line antibiotic therapy for adult medical patients

NB: Always give first dose promptly

Community acquired pneumonia

(only with consolidation on chest X-ray; document CURB-65 score)

Mild - Moderate   amoxicillin 500mg tds orally & clarithromycin* 500mg bd orally
(*MUST review at 48 hours)
(If penicillin allergy clarithromycin 500mg bd orally)

Severe: (i.e. 3 or more of CURB-65: confusion, urea>7, RR≥30, diastolic BP≤60, age≥65yr)
benzylpenicillin 1.2g qds iv & clarithromycin 500mg bd iv
(if penicillin allergy levofloxacin 500mg bd iv & clarithromycin 500mg bd iv)

ITU/HDU admission only   benzylpenicillin 1.2g qds IV & levofloxacin 500mg bd IV
Penicillin allergy: levofloxacin 500mg bd IV & clarithromycin 500mg bd IV
If urinary sepsis also likely, consider adding gentamicin 5mg/kg stat iv (max 480mg) while awaiting microbiology.

Infective exacerbation of COPD (with purulent sputum)

doxycycline 200mg stat, then 100mg od orally
OR
amoxicillin 500mg tds orally
For Type II decompensated respiratory failure – seek Respiratory advice

Simple UTI (dysuria but no systemic symptoms)

(take MSU)   trimethoprim 200mg bd orally for 3 days

UTI with systemic symptoms (fever, rigors, loin pain)

(take MSU)   co-amoxiclav 625mg tds po for 5 days plus gentamicin 5mg/kg IV stat (max 480mg)
Penicillin allergy: ciprofloxacin 500mg bd po for 5 days (must be discussed with consultant and approval documented in medical notes)

OR   If recent urological intervention, or long term urinary catheter use ertapenem 1g od IV
Review when microbiology results available

Cellulitis

Mild - Moderate   flucloxacillin 1g qds orally   (clindamycin 450mg qds orally if penicillin allergic or flucloxacillin failure)

Severe   benzylpenicillin 1.2g qds iv   (clindamycin 450mg qds iv if penicillin allergic)
PLUS
flucloxacillin 1g qds iv

NB: if rapidly progressing, +/- septic shock, severe disproportionate pain, consider necrotising fasciitis. This is a surgical emergency – seek senior and microbiology advice. Usual therapy is with meropenem and clindamycin.

Probable bacterial meningitis (must be discussed with senior medical staff)

ceftriaxone 2g bd iv

Neutropenic sepsis (neutrophils <1.0x10^9/L)

Tazocin 4.5g tds iv (discuss with SpR Haematology)
Penicillin allergy: meropenem 1g tds iv

Sever e sepsis of unknown origin

(including MEWS score of≥3; take blood cultures, then start antibiotics immediately)

amoxicillin 1g tds iv & metronidazole 500mg tds iv & gentamicin 5mg/kg stat iv (max 480mg)

For complex cases, please contact the duty microbiologist, including if the patient is recently discharged from hospital, allergy to first line regimen, infections in pregnancy

Always check for contra-indications, drug interactions and dosage modication in renal and hepatic impairment. Drugs marked in red contain penicillin.

HEART of **ENGLAND** NHS Foundation Trust

June 2008

Figure 7.1 An example of a microbiology guideline.

of antibiotics. Ideally, samples should be taken before antibiotics are given, and transported promptly to the laboratory. Whilst the identification of the causative organism will clearly not affect initial antibiotic administration, a subsequent modification to tailor treatment against a specific pathogen will not only improve efficacy but also reduce the risk of resistant strains developing in the individual patient and in the community as a whole.

Blood cultures should always be taken in the presence of sepsis or severe sepsis, without waiting for the temperature to reach an arbitrary pre-defined point. Having said this, there is some evidence

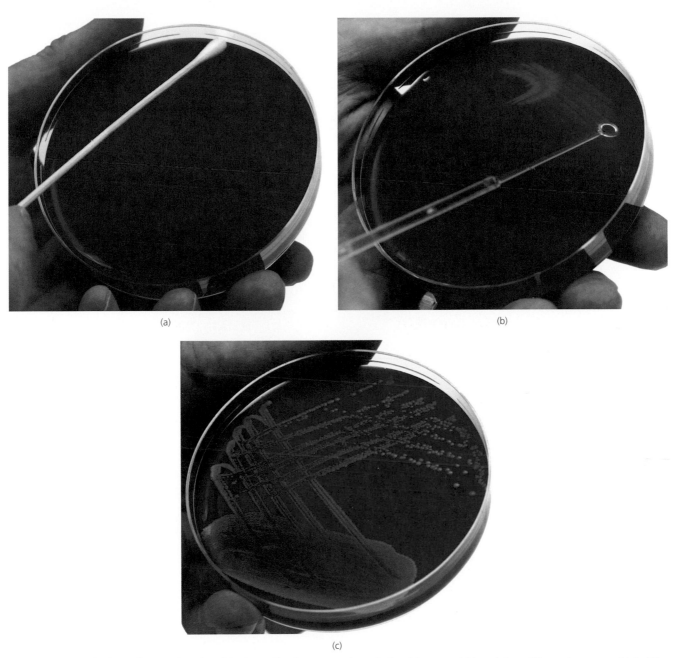

(a)

(b)

(c)

Figure 7.2 Bacterial culture of a wound swab on blood agar. The three stages shown in the pictures are: (a) inoculation of the swab over one-third of the surface of the agar; (b) spreading of any bacteria present across the surface with a sterile plastic disposable loop; and (c) the agar plate after overnight culture showing individual bacterial colonies. Reproduced with permission from McKenzie *et al*. 2009.

that sensitivity is higher if cultures are taken as the temperature is rising, and therefore consideration should be given to repeating samples if this subsequently happens. According to the presumed site or sites of infection, consideration should also be given to the sampling of urine, sputum, pus or fluid collections (including intra-abdominal and interpleural), swabs of wounds and ulcers, synovial fluid and cerebrospinal fluid.

Particularly if an intravascular device has been in place for more than 24 hours, it may be appropriate to take additional samples from the device. If a central venous catheter is a potential source of infection, then there is a case for sampling from each lumen. Multiple sampling not only increases the likelihood of isolating an

individual organism but can also help identify when the organism is a simple skin contaminant (false positive) and whether a particular device is the source of infection (Figure 7.2).

An adequate volume of blood (at least 10 ml in each bottle) is important to maximize the chances of recovery (the ability to culture colonies) of organisms. Local protocols for the correct sampling of blood cultures must be consulted and adhered to – an example of such a protocol is given in Table 7.1. False-negative blood cultures may arise from inadequate volumes of blood. Samples must be transported promptly to the microbiology laboratory for incubation, as delay can also reduce the recovery rate of organisms (Figure 7.3).

Table 7.1 Procedure for percutaneous sampling for blood culture.

- Obtain consent from the patient
- Wash your hands and adopt appropriate personal protective equipment
- Prepare sampling device (needle/syringe or vacuum collection system), anaerobic and aerobic culture bottles with plastic caps removed, two additional needles, and 2% chlorhexidine in 70% alcohol (2% CHG/70% IPA) swabs on a clean trolley
- Wash your hands again and apply gloves
- Using a disposable tourniquet, identify a suitable vein
- Clean the skin site with 2% CHG/70% IPA and allow to dry
- If using a vacuum collection device:
  - Swap the top of each bottle with a separate 2% CHG/70% IPA swab and allow to dry
  - Without repalpating the site, draw 10 ml of blood directly into each bottle
- If using a needle and syringe:
  - Without repalpating the site, sample 20 ml of blood
  - Swap the top of each bottle with a separate 2% CHG/70% IPA swab and allow to dry
  - Using a clean needle each time, inoculate each bottle with 10 ml of blood
- Label samples appropriately and transport immediately to the laboratory
- Remove gloves, wash hands and dispose appropriately of all waste

Document the procedure in the patient's notes.

CHG, chlorhexidine gluconate; IPA, isopropyl alcohol.

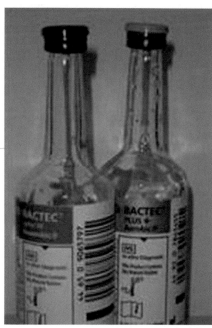

Figure 7.3 Blood culture bottles.

Additional investigations

The patient's white cell count, and differential including neutrophil count, may provide valuable additional information. However, the white cell count is neither 100% sensitive nor specific. A normal white cell count does not exclude an infective cause, and other conditions including an acute coronary syndrome can give rise to an elevated white cell count. A reduction in the white cell count over the first 12–72 hours of intervention in sepsis can provide reassurance,

just as a persistent increase may warn of failure of therapy and the need for a change in antimicrobial agent or control of the source. Beware, however, a precipitous fall in white cells, which may indicate an overwhelming infection with a failing immune response.

Other markers of systemic infection include C-reactive protein (CRP) and procalcitonin (PCT). Again, neither of these is entirely specific to sepsis, and both will rise in other conditions such as trauma. There is some evidence that PCT may exhibit a more graded response in severe sepsis – in other words, the level may more closely mirror the severity of disease.

In practice, a combination of the white cell count with either CRP or PCT in conjunction with repeated clinical assessment serves to provide a guide as to severity of disease and, with time, response to therapy.

Rapid testing using polymerase chain reaction is available for some organisms, including methicillin-resistant *Staphylococcus aureus* (MRSA), *E.coli* and group B streptococci. This near-patient method can cut the time to identification down from 48 to just a couple of hours, although it is not yet universally available.

The use of imaging to identify potential sources of sepsis is discussed in Chapter 9.

Choice of empiric antimicrobials

The use of empiric antibiotics (and antifungals) constitutes a 'best guess'. The spectrum of cover of the agents chosen should include all likely pathogens for that patient at that time. This is influenced by factors relating to the organization, to the individual patient including the co-morbidity, and to the severity of the condition.

Local antibiotic prescribing guidelines

An up-to-date local guideline, when available, should be the single most important determinant in the choice of antibiotic. An organization's Infection Control and Microbiology teams will have in-depth knowledge of the prevalence of individual organisms and their resistance profile. They may employ a policy of antibiotic rotation (periodic withdrawal of some groups of agent and reintroduction of those previously withheld) to reduce resistance. Guidelines will need to be reviewed regularly as the profile of organisms in a community changes. A good guideline (an example is given in Table 7.1) will consider some or all of the following factors. We have used the choice of antibiotic in pneumonia to illustrate some of the treatment decisions, although similar considerations will apply to all conditions.

Place of likely exposure to infecting organism

It is important to differentiate between hospital-acquired and community-acquired infections, since the likely organisms and sensitivities will vary. For example, the recommended treatment for community-acquired pneumonia (CAP) will differ from that for hospital-acquired pneumonia (HAP).

Most CAPs are due to *Streptococcus pneumoniae* or *Haemophilus influenza*. A penicillin such as amoxicillin or benzyl penicillin, in combination with a newer macrolide like clarithromycin, would therefore provide adequate cover in the majority of cases.

HAPs (pneumonias developing at least 48 hours after hospital admission), however, are rarely caused by *S. pneumoniae*, although *H. influenza* is occasionally a factor. Agents should be chosen instead to cover gram-negative bacilli such as *Pseudomonas aeruginosa*, *Klebsiella*, *Enterobacter* and *S. aureus*. This reflects the likely origin of the condition as due to microaspiration of upper airway secretions and gut contents. Recent isolates from other sources may be important in guiding therapy. Empiric therapy with a single agent has been shown to be as effective as polytherapy, and co-amoxiclav or piperacillin-tazobactam would be reasonable first-line choices.

Some organizations make a distinction between 'early' (within 5 days) and 'late' (after 5 days or more) HAPs. Again, this reflects a change in the likely pathogen profile, with *P. aeruginosa*, for example, becoming more likely. Co-amoxiclav would be less likely to have activity, and agents such as piperacillin-tazobactam or meropenem would be better choices.

Patient factors

Any history of known colonization, particularly with organisms such as MRSA, should be sought. In the case of a HAP, this may prompt treatment with an agent such as linezolid.

A history of allergy to any antibiotic should be sought and identified. The most common allergy given by a patient is to penicillins, but it should also be remembered that a true penicillin allergy carries a risk of cross-sensitivity with cephalosporins and carbapenems. Recent or recurrent use of antibiotics will increase the likelihood of resistant organisms, in which case expert advice should be sought from microbiology. In determining appropriate samples and choice of antibiotics, local guideline and policy should always be consulted.

The likely organism can be influenced by other patient factors, ranging from the simple (younger patients in the community are more commonly affected by atypical organisms such as *Mycoplasma pneumoniae* than the elderly) to complex problems such as the immunocompromised patient, who may be at risk of cytomegalovirus or *Pneumocystis carinii* infection. This special situation is discussed further in Chapter 12.

The patients' age, body mass, renal and hepatic function together with their ability to absorb via the gastrointestinal tract will all need to be taken into consideration in choosing appropriate antibiotics. For example, whilst intravenous antibiotics are strongly recommended in severe sepsis, ciprofloxacin is just as effective enterally and is easier to administer so may be chosen in patients with a functioning gut. A patient with borderline renal dysfunction carries a relative contraindication to aminoglycosides such as gentamicin. A patient with liver failure has an increased risk of fungal pneumonia, and it may be sensible to add an antifungal agent early.

Epidemics and pandemics

A cluster of cases may suggest an outbreak of *Legionella pneumophila*. The diagnosis of this condition relies on an index of suspicion and the demonstration of Legionella antigens in the urine, or identification by direct immunofluorescence or sputum culture using specialized media. Quinolones and macrolides, alone or in combination, are effective.

Mycoplasma pneumonia tends to occur in 4-yearly epidemics, but is also more prevalent in winter year on year.

A number of influenza strains can cause pneumonia and the fear of a pandemic is rife currently. Pandemic influenza is discussed in greater detail in Chapter 10. Clearly, these patients will not respond to antibiotics.

In practice, the 'best guess' will provide adequate cover in over 90% of cases. In severe sepsis, the highest dose of the appropriate agent(s) which is suitable given the patient's size and co-morbidities should be used.

Response to positive cultures

When an organism is identified from blood (or other) cultures, the possibility of contamination from the skin should first be considered. The most common contaminant is a coagulase-negative *S. aureus*. The likelihood of this organism being a contaminant is lower if it is isolated from multiple sites or at multiple times, and if the culture is positive within 12–24 hours of sampling.

If the likely source of infection is one associated with *Staphylococci*, then its significance is likely to be greater. Examples include wound and line infections, cellulitis, endocarditis, osteomyelitis and pneumonia. If line infection is suspected, then the immediate response should be to establish alternative access and remove the line. Sending its tip for culture may confirm the suspicion. Conversely, intra-abdominal sepsis is unlikely to be associated with staphylococcal infection, and it would be appropriate to continue broad-spectrum antibiotics in this context.

Organisms commonly isolated from blood cultures, with their most likely sources, are listed in Table 7.2.

Prior to full culture results becoming available, a gram stain may provide information as to the likely organism if applied to a sample containing a high yield of organisms. If the organism isolated is unlikely to be a contaminant, then antibiotics may be started empirically (if not already) based on the result of the Gram stain, or the spectrum of existing antibiotic narrowed. An example of a recommendation for first-line empiric antibiotics based on Gram

Table 7.2 Organisms commonly isolated from blood cultures and their most likely sources.

Organism from blood culture	Examples of sources
Escherichia coli	Urinary tract, intra-abdominal
Streptococcus pneumoniae	Pneumonia, meningitis
Staphylococcus aureus	Skin, soft tissue, wound, osteomyelitis, septic arthritis, pneumonia, endocarditis, intravascular devices
Streptococcus pyogenes	Cellulitis, necrotizing fasciitis
Streptococcus milleri group	Pus/abscess in lung, liver, abdomen
Coagulase-negative staphylococci	Prosthetic joint/heart valve, central line, ventriculo-peritoneal shunt
Candida albicans	Neutropaenia, abdominal surgery, central line infections

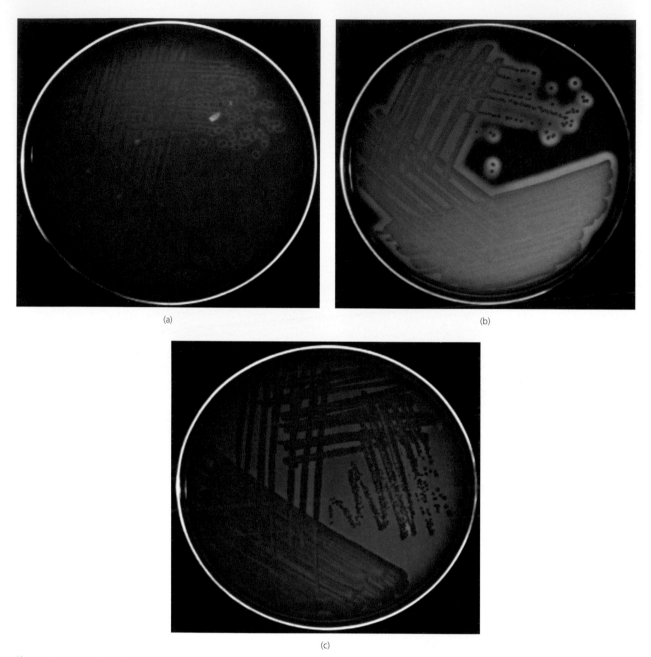

Figure 7.4 Haemolysis of blood agar by streptococci showing: (a) α-haemolysis (partial), (b) β-haemolysis (complete) and (c) no haemolysis. Reproduced with permission from McKenzie *et al.* 2009.

stain alone is given in Table 7.3, although such guidance should not replace local guidelines particularly if the source of sepsis is known. Further modification should be considered once the full identification and antibiotic sensitivities are known (Tables 7.2 and 7.3) (Figure 7.4).

De-escalation

The practice of narrowing the spectrum of cover once the causative organism and its sensitivities are identified has become known as de-escalation of therapy.

De-escalation within 48–72 hours has been shown in some studies to improve outcome for an individual patient, and in others to reduce the resistance profile of organisms in both the individual and in the population.

Not all patients with sepsis will have a causative organism found and it will not, therefore, always be possible to de-escalate therapy. However, it is good practice to set a review date at 48 hours when prescribing broad-spectrum antibiotics to prompt a review of available culture results at this time.

Persistent sepsis

If, despite appropriate antibiotic therapy, the patient is not improving or is deteriorating, the following possibilities should be considered.

Table 7.3 Recommendation for first-line empiric antibiotics based on Gram stain alone.

Gram stain result of blood culture	Suggested antibiotic(s)
Gram-negative rods – community	Cefuroxime +/− gentamicin (+/− metronidazole if anaerobe suspected) or co-amoxiclav
Gram-negative rods – hospital	Piperacillin-tazobactam or ertapenem or meropenem
Gram-positive cocci – streptococci	Benzylpenicillin (or amoxicillin if urinary or abdominal source suspected)
Gram-positive cocci – staphylococci	Flucloxacillin (or vancomycin/teicoplanin if risk factors for MRSA)
Gram-negative cocci	Ceftriaxone

MRSA, methicillin-resistant *Staphylococcus aureus*.

Continuing focus of infection – search for another fluid collection/abscess, the presence of necrotic tissue, an infected indwelling device (for example, central venous catheter), an infected prosthesis or obstruction associated with infection (biliary or renal stones).

Antibiotic resistance – consider the development of resistance in an initially sensitive isolate, or super-infection with a more resistant organism.

Host response – a vigorous host response may result in a continuation of the inflammatory response manifesting as worsening sepsis, or a lack of response (for example, the patient who is clinically deteriorating but who has a normal white cell count).

Further reading

British Thoracic Society. Guidelines for the management of community acquired pneumonia in adults. *Thorax* 2001; **56** (Suppl IV): updated 2004.

Department of Health. *Saving Lives: Taking blood cultures, a summary of best practice*, 2007. Available at www.clean-safe-care.nhs.uk

Finch RG. Empirical choice of antibiotic therapy in sepsis. *The Journal of the Royal College of Physicians of London* 2000; **34**: 528–532.

Heper Y, Akalin EH, Mistik R *et al.* Evaluation of serum C-reactive protein, procalcitonin, tumor necrosis factor alpha, and interleukin-10 levels as diagnostic and prognostic parameters in patients with community-acquired sepsis, severe sepsis, and septic shock. *European Journal of Clinical Microbiology and Infectious Diseases* 2006; **25** (8): 481–491.

McKenzie *et al. Infectious Disease: Clinical Cases Uncovered.* Blackwell Publishing, Oxford, 2009.

Shanson, DC. *Microbiology in Clinical Practice*, 3rd edn. Butterworth Heinemann, Oxford, 1999.

CHAPTER 8

Infection Prevention and Control

Fiona Lawrence, Georgina McNamara and Clare Galvin

Good Hope Hospital, Heart of England NHS Foundation Trust, Birmingham, UK

OVERVIEW

This chapter will highlight methods that have been identified in the United Kingdom with reference to international links, as a strategy to focus and streamline immediate priorities to facilitate the control and spread of infection.

- Surveillance
- Hand washing, disposal of sharps
- Uniforms, healthcare worker vaccinations
- Isolation, prudent use of antibiotics, environment
- Interventions and procedures

Introduction

Prevention of infection is now the key strategy at the forefront of the medical professions. Infection cannot be eradicated completely, since it is the price we pay for advances in medical technology and treatment. As infection rates spiral and resistance to antibiotics increase, the fundamentals of care need to be addressed.

In the United Kingdom up until 2003, infection control (IC) and prevention was very low on the political agenda. Therefore the Department of Health (DoH) document *Winning Ways* began to shape IC measures as priorities at the heart of healthcare delivery.

Awareness of IC measures is increasing, and basic knowledge improving. The message is clear, in that it is the responsibility not only of individual healthcare workers (HCWs) and cleaners but also of teams and individuals responsible for the running of healthcare systems to establish and maintain an infection prevention culture.

Florence Nightingale referred to the importance of cleanliness as far back as the 1860s. Hospitals today do not require complex systems to combat infection, rather they need to re-examine basic standards of hygiene.

Consequently, the fundamental principles to achieve infection prevention focus on education and training strategies for healthcare professionals.

ABC of Sepsis. Edited by Ron Daniels and Tim Nutbeam. © 2010 by Blackwell Publishing, ISBN: 978-1-4501-8194-5.

Surveillance

The foundation of IC is surveillance, which historically systems have consistently failed to rigorously monitor. In the United Kingdom and elsewhere, reporting systems for methicillin-resistant *Staphylococcus aureus* (MRSA) and *Clostridium difficile* (*C. difficile*) are now in use, and countries have introduced mandatory monitoring allowing a closer observation of healthcare-associated infection (HCAI).

The European Antimicrobial Resistance Surveillance System (EARRS) provides information on the occurrence and spread of antimicrobial resistance in 31 European countries. This enables countries to gain a snapshot of varying pathogens and the problems of resistance. For example, in 2006 the United Kingdom reported 3996 isolates of *S. aureus* with 42.1% being MRSA, whilst the Netherlands had 1633 reports with only 1.1% being methicillin-resistant.

All patients should have MRSA screening on admission to hospital, based on the success of the Dutch system of 'search and destroy' (Wertheim *et al.* 2004). This will enable patients to be isolated quickly following admission, thereby reducing risk to other patients in hospital. Where the Dutch system is in force, all patients identified with an HCAI are placed within single isolation rooms with *en suites*. Elsewhere, ageing hospitals with inadequate amenities may not have the capacity to achieve this standard (Box 8.1).

Box 8.1 **Future United Kingdom strategies**

- All hospitals to undergo yearly inspections based on the code of practice set down by the Health Act 2006
- If the hospitals do not meet the required standards they will be placed under special scrutiny
- By 2009 the Care Quality Commission will impose fines on poor performers
- Development of mandatory reporting of a broader range of healthcare-associated infections (HCAIs) in addition to methicillin-resistant *Staphylococcus aureus* (MRSA) and *Clostridium difficile* (*C. difficile*).
- Development of the role of inspector of microbiology in conjunction with the National Patient Safety Agency
- A public data base of infections in different counties

- Reporting of HCAI deaths and reporting serious outbreaks to the health protection agency
- Surgical site infection (SSI) surveillance (currently optional)

Latest data from the health protection agency suggests these mechanisms are achieving results, and infection rates for MRSA and *C. difficile* are on a downward trend.

Hand washing

Hand washing is the single most important measure in the prevention of HCAIs. Much education now focuses on hand washing techniques, and experience appears to support the popular view that HCWs negligently fail to maintain standards. Organizations need to examine the availability of facilities, hand hygiene agents and time. Unless these system requirements are provided then compliance with hand hygiene will remain poor. The HCW, too, must recognize the importance of hand hygiene in clinical practice.

Campaigns such as Clean Your Hands in the United Kingdom and the Clean Care is Safer Care campaign developed by the World Alliance for Patient Safety (a group which is supported by the World Health Organization or WHO) focus responsibility on the individual, the message being that the only person who can ensure your hands are clean is you. Figure 8.1 summarises current recommendations from the National Patient Safety Agency's Clean Your Hands Campaign (2009).

It is important to understand the reasons for the use of both soap and water and alcohol gels. MRSA, and a majority of bacteria, are eliminated from the hands by using alcohol hand rub, but some organisms including spores formed by *C. difficile* are not, requiring instead the washing of hands with soap and water. Hands must be decontaminated immediately before and after each and every clinical contact, with soap and water used in cases of diarrhoea or a history of *C. difficile* infection and on entering and leaving clinical areas. Alcohol gel should only be used on visibly clean hands as a minimum standard, before and after each patient contact.

Isolation

It is well documented that isolation of patients with HCAIs is beneficial in reducing transmission. However, some hospitals in England do not have sufficient facilities to individually isolate each patient with HCAI. Therefore, guidance is available to aid hospital management of this problem. Cohort nursing- caring for all patients infected with the same organism in the same ward or bay- is a reasonable alternative. This should be organized with the support of the microbiology and IC teams.

Isolation and hand washing facilities must be fit for practice. Ideally, areas should have doors rather than screens to separate from other patients. Staff should be organized to solely care of one group of patients.

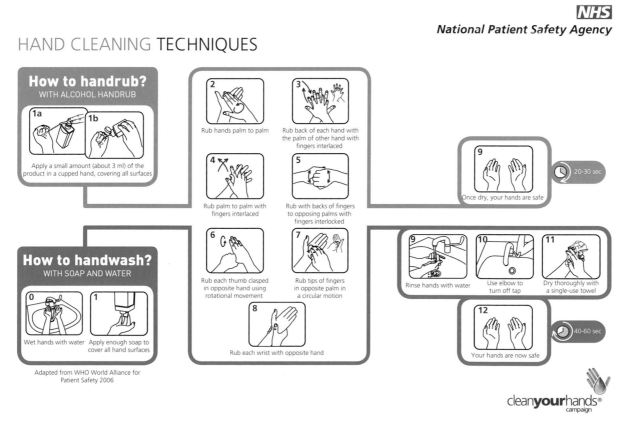

Figure 8.1 Hand cleaning techniques.

Movement of patients and staff should be kept to a minimum and only for clinical need. Where movement of patients is unavoidable, the receiving department must be made aware of IC requirements and allowed time to prepare.

Uniforms

Uniforms are unlikely to pose an IC risk, but public perception of dress standard is important. A member of the public seeing a doctor or nurse in uniform outside the workplace is unlikely to be sympathetic to the inevitability of some HCAIs.

If uniforms are laundered correctly at $60°C$, and washing machines are not overloaded, then uniforms should be 'clean'. MRSA is cleared completely at $30°C$ whilst *C. difficile* leaves around 10% of spores at $60°C$. Microbiologists confirm that this level of contamination gives no cause for concern.

Reasoning can be applied to male HCWs abandoning ties, white coats are prone to infrequent washing, and watches and cuffs of long-sleeved garments can become heavily contaminated. Similarly, any loose device such as a lanyard that may contact sequential patients should be removed. These principles have led to the general acceptance of a 'bare below the elbows' dress code.

Health worker vaccinations

Occupational health departments are responsible for ensuring that all staff are up to date with their hepatitis C, varicella, tuberculosis and influenza immunity.

WHO recommends that all HCWs should be vaccinated against influenza, and research suggests that vaccination in this group of individuals reduces mortality and morbidity amongst patients. Poor uptake to date raises questions as to the need for a higher priority for this recommendation, particularly in the context of influenza pandemics when frontline HCWs should receive vaccinations at the earliest opportunity.

Prudent use of antibiotics

It is well recognized that injudicious use of antibiotics has contributed to an increase in resistance of organisms to antibiotics. Prudent use of antibiotics does not mean neglecting to use them, as it is proven that delaying their administration in severe sepsis can increase mortality for every hour's delay. Antibiotics can be withheld, however, in some localized infections, and should certainly not be used to pacify a patient with a viral illness.

Antibiotic use should be guided by local guidelines and microbiologists, as they will have awareness of local resistance patterns and strains of organisms. Antibiotics should only be used after a treatable infection has been recognized, or if there is a high degree of suspicion of infection. It is important to identify sources immediately, so that narrow-spectrum antibiotics can be used early and broad spectrum reserved for the most resistant infections. On starting antibiotics, the dose should be individualized to the patient and the duration of therapy set.

Environment

Design of the healthcare environment is important in HCAI prevention, designing in wipe-clean surfaces, minimizing the transit of equipment and patients and reducing potential reservoirs for infection. The public expects a visibly clean environment and the standards of cleanliness are set accordingly.

In the United Kingdom, patient environment action teams (PEATs) have been assessing hospitals since 2000 and have contributed to year on year improvements in hospital cleanliness. The Healthcare Commission in the Health Act 2006 set out statutory requirements for cleanliness for the first time. Such initiatives require investment to achieve lasting change, and results of the impact of such interventions will be keenly observed.

In the United States, the systems of healthcare delivery are complex and documents do address hospital environments; however, there appears to be no statutory enforcements of standards of hygiene in hospitals. The campaign 'Saving 5 million lives' is driven by the Institute for Healthcare Improvement, and aims to reduce deaths caused by medical errors including HCAI. Submission into the programme is voluntary and not statutory. This differs from the United Kingdom's system of hospital inspections and performance tables.

Disposal of sharps

In 2003 in the United Kingdom, the National Audit Office found that needle stick injuries ranked alongside moving and handling, falls, trips and exposure to hazardous substances as the main types of accidents experienced by National Health Service (NHS) staff, presenting the HCW with an unreasonable and preventable risk of exposure to infection. Organizations should ensure that their education strategies in the safe disposal of sharps are adequate (Box 8.2).

> **Box 8.2 Minimum guidelines for the safe use of sharps bins**
> - Used sharps must be discarded into a sharps container at the point of use by the HCW
> - These must not be filled above the mark that indicates the bin is full
> - All bins for sharps should be positioned out of the reach of children at a height that enables safe disposal by all members of staff
> - They should be secured to avoid spillage

Interventions and procedures

The DoH has developed a number of high-impact interventions and adopted nationally the evidence base of the EPIC2 guidelines. Bundles of care for insertion and ongoing care of indwelling devices allow individuals to consistently carry out clinical procedures using best practice. Organisations can design education to facilitate this and monitor compliance with the guidance, allowing feedback to nurture improvement in clinical practice. Every acute hospital trust in England has signed up to this programme, focusing on the commonest sites of HCAI: urinary tract, lung, wound and blood.

The following procedures are described in detail in the *ABC of Practical Procedures*.

Aseptic no-touch technique (ANTT)

Fundamental to minimizing preventable HCAIs, the aseptic no-touch technique (ANTT) is taught at undergraduate level, but it is increasingly recognized that this requires reinforcement at the postgraduate level.

ANTT is a method used to prevent contamination of susceptible sites by microorganisms that could cause infection, by ensuring that only sterile equipment and fluids are used and the parts of components that should remain sterile, for example, the intravascular components of intravenous cannulae, are not touched or allowed to come into contact with non-sterile surfaces.

Blood cultures

It is estimated that contamination of samples occurs in approximately 10% of all blood culture collections, giving false results leading to inaccurate reporting of HCAI and potential for inappropriate treatment (Box 8.3).

Box 8.3 **Appropriate practice in the sampling of blood cultures**

- Blood cultures should be taken whenever a systemic infection or bacteraemia is suspected, irrespective of temperature
- They should be repeated if the patient subsequently 'spikes' a temperature (higher rate of capture of organisms)
- The appropriate aseptic technique should always be used
- Once taken, cultures should be transported immediately to the laboratory incubator
- If indwelling vascular access catheters have been in place for more than 24 hours, samples should be taken percutaneously and from each device

---

Peripheral venous cannulae (PVCs)

In the United Kingdom there are over 6 million hospital admissions per year. It is estimated that 80–90% of patients admitted to hospital have a peripheral venous cannulae (PVC) sited at least once, with an estimated bacteraemia rate per insertion of 0.3–1%. The need for careful placement is often neglected and their contribution to HCAIs undervalued.

Only trained and competent staff using strict ANTT should carry out intravenous cannula insertion. The number of devices attached (such as three-way taps and extensions) will be kept to the absolute minimum consistent with clinical need.

Insertion sites should be regularly inspected for signs of infection and the cannula removed if infection is suspected. They will be kept in place for the minimum time necessary and changed every 72 hours irrespective of the presence of infection. Staff should document the date of insertion and date of removal of the device

routinely. This helps establish clear monitoring and audit systems, and enables surveillance through root cause analysis in the event of an HCAI resulting.

Visual Infusion Phlebitis Score

The Visual Infusion Phlebitis (VIP) score is a tool developed to promote review of indwelling devices with regard to signs of local infection. It is recommended that it be applied and recorded for each indwelling at least every 8 hours (Box 8.4). ANTT should be employed for ongoing care including port injections, and dressing changes. A solution of 2% chlorhexidine gluconate in 70% isopropyl alcohol is recommended and should be allowed to dry. An occlusive, transparent dressing should be applied to ensure visibility of the site.

Administration sets will be changed immediately following a blood transfusion, and every 24 hours if used for intravenous feed. For other clear fluids, change will occur at 72 hours.

Once an administration set is disconnected, it should not be reconnected.

Box 8.4 **Visual Infusion Phlebitis (VIP) scoring system. Adapted with permission from Andrew Jackson**

Signs	Score	Action
IV site appears healthy	0	**No signs of phlebitis** OBSERVE CANNULA
One of the following is evident: • Slight pain near IV site Or • Slight redness near IV site	1	Possibly first signs of phlebitis OBSERVE CANNULA
Two of the following are evident: • Pain at IV site • Erythema • Swelling	2	Early stage of phlebitis RESITE CANNULA
All of the following signs are evident: • Pain along path of cannula • Erythema • Induration	3	Medium stages of Phlebitis RESITE CANNULA CONSIDER TREATMENT
All of the following signs are evident and extensive: • Pain along path of cannula • Erythema • Induration • Palpable venous cord	4	Advanced stages of phlebitis or the start of thrombophlebitis RESITE CANNULA CONSIDER TREATMENT
All of the following signs are evident and extensive: • Pain along path of cannula • Erythema • Induration • Palpable venous cord • Pyrexia	5	Advanced stages of thrombophlebitis INITIATE TREATMENT RESITE CANNULA

Feeding lines

Intravenous feeding lines (parenteral nutrition) are used when there is no suitable alternative, and then kept in place for as short a time as possible. A dedicated single lumen line (preferred) or lumen of a multichannel line should be used. No other infusion or injection should go via this route. Any additives to intravenous fluid containers should be introduced aseptically in a unit or safety cabinet designed for the purpose, by trained staff using strictly aseptic techniques.

Central venous catheters (CVCs)

Central venous catheter (CVC) insertion, manipulation and removal should be undertaken by trained and competent staff using strictly aseptic techniques. The subclavian route is associated with the lowest risk of infection. CVCs carry an associated bacteraemia rate of approximately 8%, with additive risk the longer the line is in situ. CVCs should only be used when clinical need outweighs risk and removed as soon as possible.

Urinary catheters

Urinary catheters will be used when there is no suitable alternative, and kept in place for as short a time as possible. Where long-term indwelling use is unavoidable, a catheter of low allergenicity will be used.

Urinary catheter insertion, manipulation, washing out, urine sampling and removal will be undertaken by trained and competent staff using strictly aseptic techniques. Patients and carers will be educated in catheter maintenance with an emphasis on personal hygiene.

The date of insertion and date of removal of the device will be documented in the clinical record as a matter of routine.

Personal protective equipment (PPE)

This relates to the protection of the HCW from bodily fluids. Gloves should be used for all invasive procedures and all activities that have been assessed as carrying a risk of exposure to blood, body fluids, secretions and excretions. Gloves may provide a false sense of security with regard to infection prevention and the integrity of these is not absolute; therefore, it remains imperative that excellent hand hygiene must be adhered to before and after use. The individual should decide on surgical or examination gloves on the basis of the procedure they are undertaking.

Aprons should be treated as single-use items. Disposable plastic aprons must be worn when there is a risk that clothing may become contaminated with pathogenic microorganisms or blood, body fluids, secretions or excretions.

Face masks and eye protection must be worn where there is a risk of body fluids splashing into the face and eyes. In addition, respiratory protective equipment, (for example, a particulate filter mask), must be used when recommended for the care of patients with respiratory infections transmitted by airborne particles. These

facilities are only just filtering down to the HCW and much education and training is still required.

Conclusion

This section only covers the tip of the iceberg with regard to available guidance for clinical procedures; therefore, referral to relevant local guidelines is advised.

The importance of the prevention of infection cannot be stressed enough, and it must be noted that key documents listed within this chapter will be revised and superseded; therefore, it is the responsibility of every HCW to maintain awareness of current guidance.

Useful websites

clean your hands campaign www.npsa.nhs.uk/cleanyourhands
PEAT inspections www.npsa.nhs.uk/peat
The European Antimicrobial Resistance Surveillance System http://www.rivm.nl/earss/
The Health Protection Agency http://www.hpa.org.uk/
Institute for Health Care Improvement – Saving 5 million lives. http://www.ihi.org/IHI/Programs/Campaign/
National Audit Office http://www.nao.org.uk/publications/other_publications.htm
Clean Care Safer Care http://www.who.int/patientsafety/events/05/global_challenge/en/index.html

Further reading

Department of Health. *Getting Ahead of the Curve. A Strategy for Combating Infectious Diseases* (including other aspects of health protection). DH, London, 2002. Available from: http://www.dh.gov.uk/assetRoot/04/06/08/75/04060875.pdf [Accessed 28th August 2006].
Department of Health. *Winning Ways: Working Together to Reduce Health Care Associated Infection in England*, Report from the Chief Medical Officer. DH, London, 2003. Available from: http://www.dh.gov.uk/assetRoot/04/06/46/89/04064689.pdf [Accessed 28th August 2006].
Department of Health. *Towards Cleaner Hospitals and Lower Rates of Infection: A Summary of Action*. DH, London, 2004. Available from: http://www.dh.gov.uk/assetRoot/04/08/58/61/04085861.pdf [Accessed 28th August 2006].
Department of Health. *Saving Lives: A Delivery Programme to Reduce Health Care Associated Infection (HCAI) Including MRSA*. DH, London, 2005. Available from: http://www.dh.gov.uk/PolicyAndGuidance/HealthAndSocialCareTopics/HealthcareAcquiredInfection/HealthcareAcquiredGeneralInformation/SavingLivesDeliveryProgramme/fs/en [Accessed 28th August 2006].
Department of Health. *Essential Steps to Safe, Clean Care: Reducing Health Care Associated Infection*. DH, London, 2006. http://www.dh.gov.uk/PolicyAndGuidance/HealthAndSocialCareTopics/HealthcareAcquiredInfection/HealthcareAcquiredGeneralInformation/SavingLivesDeliveryProgramme/fs/en [Accessed 28th August 2006].
Department of Health. *The Health Act 2006. Code of Practice for the Prevention and Control of Healthcare Associated Infections*. DOH, London, 2006. Available from: http://www.dh.gov.uk/assetRoot/04/13/93/37/04139337.pdf [Accessed 28th August 2006].
Department of Health. *Uniforms and Workwear: An Evidence Base for Developing Local Policy*. DOH, London, 2007. Available from: http://www.dh.

gov.uk/en/Publicationsandstatistics/Publications/ PublicationsPolicyAndGuidance/DH_078433 [Accessed 28th August 2006].

Department of Health. *Clean, Safe Care: Reducing Infections and Saving Lives.* DOH, London, 2008.

Jackson A. A battle in the vein: infusion phlebitis. *Nursing Times* 1998; **94** (4): 68–71.

NHS Estates. A Matron's Charter: An Action Plan for Cleaner Hospitals, 2004. Available from: http://www.dh.gov.uk/assetRoot/04/09/15/07/04091507. pdf [Accessed 28th August 2006].

Pratt RJ, Pellowe CM, Wilson JA, Loveday H P, Harper PJ Jones SRLJ. Epic 2: national evidence-based guidelines for preventing healthcare-associated infections in NHS hospitals in England. *Journal of Hospital Infection* 2007; **65**: S1–S31.

Wertheim HFL, Vos MC, Boelens HAM *et al.* Low prevalence of methicillin-resistant Staphylococcus aureus (MRSA) at hospital admission in the Netherlands: the value of search and destroy and restrictive antibiotic use. *Journal of Hospital Infection* 2004; **56** (4): 321–325.

CHAPTER 9

The Role of Imaging in Sepsis

Morgan Cleasby

Good Hope Hospital, Heart of England NHS Foundation Trust, Birmingham, UK

OVERVIEW

- Modern imaging techniques are important in locating the source of sepsis

- A chest radiograph (CXR) remains an important baseline investigation

- Ultrasound is quick, safe and can be portable. It is the first-line investigation for the biliary, renal and gynaecological tracts, and may show intra-abdominal abscesses. It may be difficult in obese patients

- Computerized tomography (CT) is better at showing the bowel and retroperitoneum, and is the investigation of choice in patients following abdominal surgery. It also shows intrapulmonary and intracranial abscesses. However, it involves a high dose of radiation

- Magnetic resonance imaging (MRI) is the modality of choice for spinal imaging and shows more subtle intracranial pathology than CT. It is also used for imaging osteomyelitis. However, it is not suitable for unstable patients and there are a number of contraindications

- Image-guided techniques are important for diagnostic aspiration and therapeutic drainage of abscesses and infected hollow viscera

---

Introduction

In the patient with sepsis, history taking and examination will suggest the likely source in many cases. Imaging may help to confirm the primary site or to search for it if not clinically apparent. This chapter will discuss the various imaging modalities used to assess the likely site of origin of septic illness, including their relative strengths and weaknesses. Interventional radiological techniques will also be discussed, including diagnostic aspiration and therapeutic percutaneous drainage of abscesses or infected hollow viscera.

Whenever sepsis is suspected clinically, this should be highlighted to the radiologist when requesting imaging investigations. This will enable the appropriate examination to be performed, within a

suitably urgent timeframe. It is recommended that indices of the severity of sepsis should be included in the radiological referral, such as the white cell count, evidence of raised inflammatory markers and evidence of renal impairment, particularly if iodinated intravenous contrast is likely to be used. If the patient is critically ill, the critical care team should be consulted in order to ensure that an appropriate level of support is available whilst the patient attends the imaging department.

Modalities

Table 9.1 gives an overview of the imaging modalities that can be used in the investigation of sepsis. These techniques will be discussed in turn.

Plain radiography

The usefulness of plain radiographic examination should not be overlooked. A chest radiograph (CXR) should be considered a first-line investigation when a patient presents with sepsis. It may show the primary source of sepsis (such as pneumonic consolidation, pleural empyema or pulmonary abscess), or secondary

Table 9.1 Major indications for the different imaging modalities in sepsis.

Modality	Principal indications
Plain radiography	CXR: Lungs, pleura, mediastinum
	AXR: Renal calculi, often superseded by ultrasound or CT
Ultrasound	Abdomen/pelvis: Biliary, renal, gynaecological abscesses
	Thorax: Pleural collections
CT	Abdomen/pelvis: Bowel, retroperitoneum
	Post-operative
	Chest: Lung abscesses, mediastinum
	Head: Cerebral, extradural abscesses
	Sinuses, mastoids
MRI	Brain: As per CT
	Spine: Extradural abscesses, discitis
	Bone: Osteomyelitis
Nuclear medicine	White cell scan: Occult source of infection
	Gallium scan: Pyrexia of unknown origin

CXR, chest radiograph; AXR, abdominal radiograph; CT, computerized tomography; MRI, magnetic resonance imaging.

ABC of Sepsis. Edited by Ron Daniels and Tim Nutbeam. © 2010 by Blackwell Publishing, ISBN: 978-1-4501-8194-5.

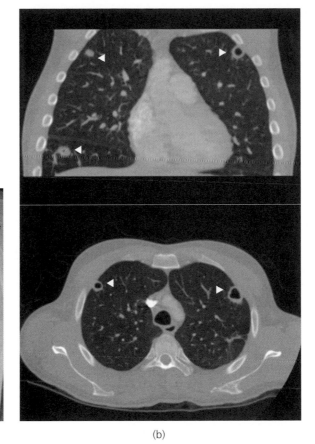

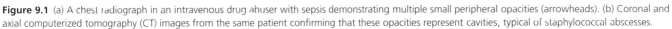

Figure 9.1 (a) A chest radiograph in an intravenous drug abuser with sepsis demonstrating multiple small peripheral opacities (arrowheads). (b) Coronal and axial computerized tomography (CT) images from the same patient confirming that these opacities represent cavities, typical of staphylococcal abscesses.

signs. Examples of the latter include left atrial enlargement and pulmonary oedema secondary to mitral valve incompetence from infective endocarditis, or an elevated hemidiaphragm and basal atelectasis secondary to a subphrenic abscess. Multiple peripheral lung cavities may suggest the haematogenous spread of staphylococcal sepsis from a peripheral superficial abscess, or the possibility of intravenous drug abuse (Figure 9.1).

Other radiographic examinations have more specific indications: plain abdominal radiographs (AXRs) are high- dose examinations, equivalent to up to 35 CXRs and should only be requested by senior clinicians if they are likely to alter management. If an abdominal ultrasound or computerized tomography (CT) examination is to be requested, the AXR need not be performed. An AXR may be useful to consider the presence of renal calculi in urological sepsis, although not all calculi are radio-opaque, and these patients are likely to require an ultrasound or CT scan of the renal tract. The presence of air in the biliary tree (pneumobilia) raises the possibility of biliary sepsis (Figure 9.2) although the most common cause nowadays is a previous sphincterotomy. Portal venous gas secondary to massive intra-abdominal sepsis is highly likely to be an antemortem finding.

Plain radiographs will show bone destruction at sites of osteomyelitis, or vertebral end-plate destruction in the spine in discitis, although magnetic resonance imaging (MRI) is much more sensitive to early changes in these conditions.

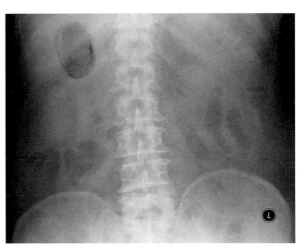

Figure 9.2 A plain abdominal radiograph showing gas in the wall of the gallbladder in the right upper quadrant in a diabetic patient with sepsis and right upper quadrant pain: the diagnosis is emphysematous cholecystitis.

Ultrasound

Ultrasound is a powerful imaging technique, which is readily available, quick and offers a high spatial resolution. It is excellent in distinguishing fluid collections from solid masses and can be used to guide interventions. It is also a portable technique, which can be utilized in sick patients, for example, in the intensive care unit. It

Table 9.2 Advantages and disadvantages of ultrasound as a modality for the investigation of sepsis.

Ultrasound

Advantages	Disadvantages
No ionizing radiation	Operator dependent
Quick	Patient dependent
Readily available	Difficult in obese patients
Portable	Unable to visualize behind bony or air interfaces – may fail to demonstrate gas-containing abscesses
Good for solid organs	
Demonstrates fluid	
Good in slim patients	

has disadvantages, however, in that it is highly operator and patient dependent. It requires technical and interpretative skills on behalf of the operator. Views are usually excellent in a slim, compliant and mobile patient. Patients who are obese, agitated, confused, in pain or immobile may be a challenge to image effectively (Table 9.2).

Ultrasound is the first-line investigation for considering sepsis in the biliary tree and urinary tract. Biliary dilatation and the presence of biliary calculi are readily assessed. Hydronephrosis and hydroureter are similarly well demonstrated with ultrasound (Figure 9.3). Intra-abdominal collections can be demonstrated with ultrasound although note that gas-filled bowel loops may obscure the presence of abscesses between them, or retroperitoneal disease. Similarly, gas-containing abscesses can be misinterpreted as normal bowel loops. It should be remembered that intraperitoneal abscesses tend to lie in the most dependent parts of the peritoneal cavity such as the pouch of Douglas or rectovesical fossa. A full bladder is required to visualize the pelvis in order to displace the bowel loops which otherwise may obscure views.

Ultrasound may show a necrotic pancreas in pancreatitis, appendix masses and pericolic diverticular abscesses. However these cannot be excluded if not seen: if clinical suspicion remains high, CT is indicated.

Ultrasound is the modality of choice for imaging the gynaecological tract. Pelvic inflammatory disease, pyosalpinx and pyometria (pus in the Fallopian tubes and uterine cavity respectively) can be

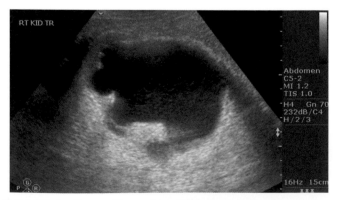

Figure 9.3 An ultrasound image of a grossly hydronephrotic kidney. Specular internal echoes within the fluid raise the possibility of pyonephrosis. In the context of sepsis, urgent nephrostomy is required.

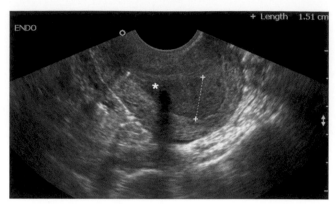

Figure 9.4 A transvaginal ultrasound image of the uterus in a patient with an intrauterine contraceptive device (IUCD) in situ and a foul-smelling vaginal discharge. The endometrial cavity is distended by reflective pus (pyometria), as measured at 1.5 cm. The IUCD causes an acoustic shadow in the image (*).

demonstrated (Figure 9.4). If the urinary bladder is empty or views are incomplete, transvaginal scanning allows the probe to be placed close to the area of interest (unless there is an intact hymen).

Ultrasound is useful in other body systems also. It is a good modality for assessing the pleural space and helps differentiate between solid pleural thickening and fluid when a CXR shows pleural opacification. Ultrasound is better than CT at demonstrating the presence of septations within pleural collections. Biconvexity of shape and the presence of internal echoes suggest the presence of empyema rather than a serous parapneumonic collection. Echocardiography is used to image the heart, though in the United Kingdom it is usually performed by cardiologists rather than radiologists. It is indicated to consider the presence of vegetations on the cardiac valves, if infective endocarditis is suspected, particularly if there is evidence of multiple systemic septic emboli.

Ultrasound may be used to look for joint infusions if septic arthritis is suspected and may help characterize soft tissue masses and abscesses.

Computerized tomography

The diagnostic power of CT has taken a massive leap forward in recent years due to the development of the latest generation multi-slice scanners. CT is no longer primarily an axial imaging modality. Images can be reconstructed in sagittal, coronal and oblique planes, and three-dimensional image displays can be produced. It is becoming a first-line imaging investigation in the investigation of many acute abdominal conditions. It has strengths over ultrasound in better demonstrating the retroperitoneum and giving more complete visualization of the bowel. Intra-abdominal adiposity can aid diagnosis in CT as it separates the organs and bowel loops: increased density within the fat planes can be a marker of inflammation (Table 9.3).

It should be remembered, however, that CT examinations administer a high dose of ionizing radiation to the patient, up to the equivalent of 500 CXRs, and therefore imaging modalities that avoid ionizing radiation should be used wherever possible, especially in young patients. Also, there is a small risk of adverse reaction to intravenous iodinated contrast agents that are likely to be used

Table 9.3 Advantages and disadvantages of computerized tomography (CT) as a modality for the investigation of sepsis.

CT

Advantages	Disadvantages
Quick	High dose of ionizing radiation
Readily available	Risk of IV contrast (especially in diabetics and in pre-existent renal impairment)
Multiplanar on modern scanners	Demonstrates density, but not fluid state
Good for lungs, bowel, retroperitoneum	May fail to show septations/loculations
Intra-abdominal fat can be useful	May fail to show biliary calculi

IV, intravenous.

in considering the presence of infection. The risk of severe anaphylactoid reaction is as low as 0.01%. However, contrast-induced nephrotoxicity is a more common adverse reaction particularly in those with pre-existent renal impairment and/or diabetes mellitus. A list of indications and contraindications for the use of such contrast is given in Box 8.1.

Box 9.1 Indications and contraindications for the use of iodinated contrast in CT in sepsis

Area	Principal indications
CT head	To consider abscess, extradural empyema or meningeal enhancement
	Useful if suspicion of secondary venous sinus thrombosis
CT thorax	Not necessary to demonstrate consolidation or pulmonary abscess
	Useful for pleural disease or to assess mediastinal nodes
CT abdomen/ pelvis	Invariably indicated to best assess the liver, spleen and pancreas
	Oral contrast is also useful to differentiate bowel loops from abscesses
	Uncontrasted CT of the renal tract is used if the clinical question is solely to question the presence of calculi

Contraindications

Absolute: Previous severe reaction to iodinated contrast
Relative: History of unstable asthma or atopy
Renal impairment (glomerular filtration rate <30 ml/minute)
• especially if diabetic, hypertensive, on nephrotoxic drugs
• clinical urgency might outweigh risks
• haemofiltration can be used to clear contrast in severe renal impairment
Previous mild reaction to iodinated contrast

Abdominal CT is a very useful examination in detecting abdominal collections for reasons cited above. It is especially useful in post-operative patients with suspected intra-abdominal collections

when pain, dressings and gas-containing bowel loops from the ileus may hinder the use of ultrasound. CT of the thorax is sometimes used in the further delineation of intrapulmonary abscesses or pleural empyemas (Figure 9.5), particularly if thoracic surgery is being considered. CT head scanning is not routinely indicated in uncomplicated cases of meningitis, and obtaining a scan should not delay giving the first dose of antibiotics. Head scanning is indicated if there is decreased conscious level, focal neurology or papilloedema, in order to exclude a space-occupying lesion prior to lumbar puncture. If there is any clinical suspicion of sinus disease or mastoiditis, a head scan is indicated to consider the presence of an extradural abscess (Figure 9.5). Head scanning is also indicated if there is a penetrating head injury, open skull fracture or previous neurosurgery that could give rise to intracranial sepsis.

Magnetic resonance imaging

MRI has advantages over CT in that it has excellent soft tissue contrast, which makes it a more sensitive neurological imaging modality. Gadolinium enhancement is used in looking for infective illness. It is more sensitive than CT in looking for diffuse meningeal enhancement in meningitis. This may be important to assess in chronic basal meningitis when atypical organisms, including mycobacteria, need to be considered. Gadolinium-enhanced MRI is also the modality of choice for spinal imaging, and should be requested if an extradural abscess in the spinal canal or a discitis is suspected (Figure 9.6).

Other advantages of MRI include the absence of ionizing radiation, but there are a number of disadvantages and contraindications (Table 9.4): the examinations can be lengthy, for which the patient needs to lie still in a confined and noisy space. Access to the patient is limited, and this is not the ideal environment for an unstable patient. MRI is contraindicated in the presence of cardiac pacemakers, intraorbital metallic foreign bodies and a number of prostheses or intracranial aneurysm clips.

As in neuroimaging, the excellent soft tissue contrast makes MRI the best modality for demonstrating marrow oedema and thus for considering the presence and extent of osteomyelitis. However, ultrasound and CT are much more likely to be used by radiologists in the imaging of sepsis than MRI, other than in these roles mentioned.

Table 9.4 Advantages and disadvantages of magnetic resonance imaging (MRI) as a modality for the investigation of sepsis.

MRI

Advantages	Disadvantages
Avoids ionizing radiation	Lengthy examinations
Multiplanar	Availability has historically been limited
Excellent soft tissue contrast	Patient compliance (claustrophobia)
Good for neuroaxis, bone marrow, soft tissues	Numerous contraindications including pacemakers, certain prostheses, loose metal fragments
	Enclosed magnet bore, limited access to patients (not suitable for unstable patients)

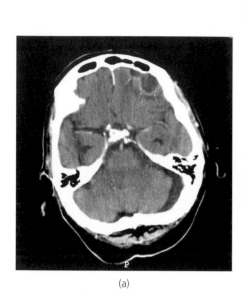

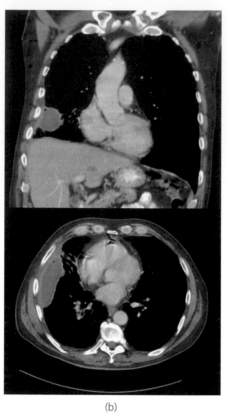

Figure 9.5 (a) Contrasted axial computerized tomography (CT) of the head shows a biconvex low-density collection with rim enhancement (arrows) in the left frontal region representing an extradural empyema in this patient with sepsis. (b) In the same patient, axial and coronal reformats of CT of the thorax reveal the primary source of infection – a pleural empyema containing a pocket of gas seen laterally in the right hemithorax. The coronal section demonstrates the convex medial border indenting the lung, a feature that will be seen on the chest radiograph (CXR) also.

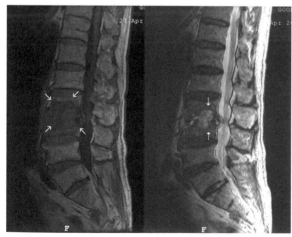

Figure 9.6 From left to right, T1-weighted and T2-weighted sagittal magnetic resonance imaging (MRI) of the lumbar spine showing an infective discitis of the L2–L3 disc. Low-signal oedema is seen in the vertebral bodies either side of the disc on the T1-weighted image (arrows), high signal pus is seen in the disc space on the T2-weighted image, with destruction of the vertebral endplate on either side (dotted arrows). The infected disc bulges posteriorly to compress the lumbar thecal sac.

Nuclear medicine

The use of nuclear medicine in the search for an unknown source of sepsis or pyrexial illness has diminished with the technological advances made in cross-sectional imaging techniques in recent years. There is still some advantage in the use of labelled white cell scanning to track down elusive sites of sepsis. Gallium scanning can be used for a similar purpose, and as there is increased uptake in tumour cells, can be used for pyrexia of unknown origin when the differential diagnosis may lie between infection and neoplastic conditions such as lymphoma.

Interventional radiology

Percutaneous techniques under imaging guidance can be utilized for the diagnostic sampling of infected structures or collections in order to isolate causative organisms and check antibiotic sensitivities. Percutaneous drains can be placed in order to drain abscesses or infected collections in a variety of anatomical locations (Figure 9.7). Ultrasound, CT, fluoroscopy and even MRI can be used as the guiding modalities, dependent on the site of infection, availability and user preference. Trochar techniques or initial needle puncture followed by a Seldinger technique over a guidewire can be used to site a drainage catheter (Figure 9.8).

The possibility of a pyonephrosis in an obstructed kidney is a medical emergency requiring urgent percutaneous nephrostomy and these patients are often potentially unstable due to the possibility of gram-negative sepsis. Similarly, suppurative cholangitis may require urgent percutaneous transhepatic biliary drainage. An

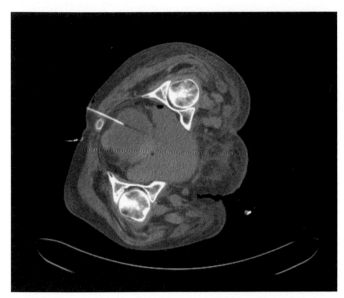

Figure 9.7 Computerized tomography (CT)-guided drainage of a pelvic collection in the rectovesical fossa, performed in a decubitus position. A line of puncture close to the lateral aspect of the lower sacrum or coccyx is chosen to avoid the neurovascular structures in the sciatic foramen.

acutely inflamed gallbladder can be drained percutaneously if a patient is too unwell from overwhelming sepsis to tolerate a definitive surgical procedure. The radiologist will usually request to see that there are an adequate number of platelets and no coagulopathy prior to performing such procedures. Success rates of 90% are seen on draining simple abscesses. It should be noted that a patient who is not overtly septic at the time of percutaneous drainage might become so periprocedurally. Thus, the patient should have commenced antibiotic therapy prior to drainage. Complications including development of septic shock, haemorrhage and bowel perforation are described in between 3 and 10% of cases.

> Imaging can add diagnostic value, and guide definitive therapy, when used in conjunction with clinical assessment and laboratory investigations.

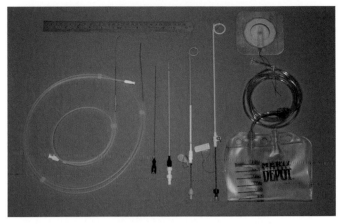

Figure 9.8 A selection of puncture needles, guidewires and drainage catheters used in the percutaneous drainage of abscesses. Thick pus may require the placement of a catheter of up to 12-French diameter (4 mm).

Acknowledgement

We thank Dr Sara Williams for supplying images for Figures 9.4 and 9.5.

Further reading

Cox PH & Buscombe JR. *The Imaging of Infection and Inflammation.* Kluwer Academic Publishers, The Netherlands, 1998.

Dawson P. Adverse reactions to intravascular contrast agents. *British Medical Journal* 2006; **333** (7570): 675.

Lee MJ. Non-traumatic abdominal emergencies: imaging and intervention in sepsis. *European Radiology* 2004; **12** (9): 2172–2179.

Mcdowell RK & Dawson SL. Evaluation of the abdomen in sepsis of unknown origin. *Radiologic Clinics of North America* 1996; **34** (1): 177–190.

Smith TP, Ryan JM & Niklason LE. Sepsis in the interventional radiology patient. *Journal of Vascular and Interventional Radiology* 2004; **15** (4): 317–325.

The Royal College of Radiologists. *Making the Best Use of Clinical Radiology Services: Referral Guidelines*, 6th edn. The Royal College of Radiologists, London, 2007.

CHAPTER 10

Presentations in Medical Patients

Nandan Gautam

University Hospitals Birmingham, Birmingham, UK

OVERVIEW

- Medical causes of sepsis are common
- The general care of the medical patient with sepsis is the same as for any other patient with sepsis
- Urinary tract infections (UTIs) remain the most frequent cause of healthcare-associated infection (HCAI)
- Pneumonia accounts for up to 60% of cases of severe sepsis
- Line-related infections are an important preventable source of severe sepsis
- Bacterial meningitis accounts for a small proportion of cases of severe sepsis but can be rapidly fatal

Introduction

The medical patient with sepsis is a very common occurrence and can present in a wide variety of ways. The most common and serious categories of infection will be considered here. It must be remembered that any hospitalized patient can develop any form of infection but patterns do exist and so a standardized approach to resuscitation (Box 10.1) and empirical treatment should be followed. Only by careful history taking, examination and timely investigations will the appropriate information and positive microbiology be available to guide ongoing treatment.

Box 10.1 Standardized approach to any patient with sepsis

1. Perform **A**irway, **B**reathing, **C**irculation, **D**isability, **E**xposure (ABCDE) assessment, initiate immediate therapy

   May include: Clinical assessment
   Airway support
   High-flow oxygen
   Cannulation
   Fluid challenges
   Urine output monitoring

   Blood glucose measurement
   Temperature regulation

2. Cross check to ensure that the following have been performed:

   High-flow oxygen therapy
   Cannulation
   Fluid challenges if circulation compromised
   Urine output monitoring

3. Perform diagnostics specific to sepsis:

   May include: Cultures (blood and others)
   Lactate measurement
   Haemoglobin and other blood tests
   Imaging to identify source

4. Complete therapies specific to sepsis:
   IV broad-spectrum antibiotics:
   Control source of infection

Rapid initial assessment using the ABCDE approach. The "Sepsis Six"

1. Give high flow oxygen (via non-rebreathe mask)
2. Take blood cultures
3. Give broad-spectrum IV antibiotics
4. Start IV fluid resuscitation
5. Check haemoglobin and lactate
6. Place and monitor urinary catheter

Throughout this book, suggestions for appropriate antibiotics are presented as a guide only. Local microbiology guidelines and advice should be followed.

Urinary tract infections (UTIs)

Urinary tract infections (UTIs) are very common, and most are self-limiting or require a short course of oral antibiotics only. However, susceptible patients can present with systemic upset and even septic shock. The patient with sepsis secondary to a UTI will often have involvement of the proximal urinary tract and may have a pyelonephritis.

ABC of Sepsis. Edited by Ron Daniels and Tim Nutbeam. © 2010 by Blackwell Publishing, ISBN: 978-1-4501-8194-5.

Diagnosis

The dipstick is a useful test of exclusion. The absence of both leukocytes (an esterase test indicating white cell activity) and nitrites (consequence of bacterial activity) virtually excludes a bacterial infection. The red cell indicator may point to a glomerulonephritis or ureteric stones. A positive dipstick, however, does not confirm the presence of a UTI as false positives are common – a careful history and examination remain important.

Urine should be sent for microbiology only if the patient is unwell and has a positive dipstick assay.

Treatment
Community-acquired without systemic symptoms
Amoxicillin is no longer an acceptable first-line agent as there is increasing resistance. Alternatives are co-amoxiclav or trimethoprim as first-line and carbapenems, piperacillin/tazobactam or quinolones as second-line therapy. Nitrofurantoin is rapidly excreted by normal kidneys and is concentrated in the urine, so is less useful in patients with systemic features where bacteraemia is likely. Cephalosporins and quinolones are increasingly avoided due to the association with Clostridium difficile infection, but do have a role in pregnancy where they are thought to be safer. Treatment is commonly for 1–5 days.

Hospital-acquired or with systemic symptoms
UTIs are the most common hospital-acquired infections. The biggest risk factor for this is urinary catheterization. The risk of developing a bacteriuria (presence of bacteria in the urine) is around 5–7% per day a catheter is in situ, and around one-third of patients with bacteriuria will have symptoms of a UTI. However, asymptomatic detection of bacteria in the urine must be regarded with caution as catheters frequently become colonized with bacteria and with candida and this does not imply infection. In addition to community-acquired organisms, staphylococci including methicillin-resistant *Staphylococcus aureus* (MRSA), pseudomonas and *candida* should be considered. Hospitalized patients are also more likely to be infected with extended spectrum beta lactamase (ESBL)-producing organisms.

Treatment requires the removal of any catheter, if at all possible, and the use of antibiotics such as ciprofloxacin or carbapenems if ESBL producers are likely. Because local resistance patterns will vary hugely, urine microbiology and culture should be carried out and microbiology advice sought as soon as practical.

UTIs may indicate structural lesions. Renal tract imaging is advised if UTIs occur frequently in women, after one or two episodes in men or if there are other features of renal tract involvement such as haematuria or red cell casts.

Pyelonephritis

Symptoms suggestive of pyelonephritis include loin or flank pain and tenderness, pyrexia and rigors, and nausea and vomiting. Susceptible patients include those with diabetes and those with recurrent infections, structural abnormality or stones. Within these patient groups those with indwelling catheters are at further risk.

Treatment

Definitive antibiotic treatment will be guided by blood and urine cultures. Acute empirical therapy should be with an agent that covers common pathogens, has a high level of systemic availability and can be given intravenously (IV). Ciprofloxacin, cefuroxime or gentamicin are all reasonable choices. Of these, ciprofloxacin is often the most appropriate as the patient can be switched to its oral form as soon as nausea and vomiting settle. Local bacterial ecology must be considered and microbiology guidelines followed.

The renal tract must be imaged to look for structural abnormalities, perinephric or parenchymal abscesses. These may require drainage using a percutaneous approach by a urologist or an interventional radiologist.

Skin, soft tissue and bone infections

Cellulitis (Figure 10.1) is an inflammatory condition affecting the dermis and subcutaneous tissues. Typically, gram-positive organisms locally invade damaged skin and the resultant inflammatory state leads to characteristic pain, erythema, local oedema and linear demarcation.

Cellulitis is very common and accounts for around 5–10% of referrals to hospital; there is an increased incidence in those with diabetes, steroid users and patients with vascular insufficiency. Cellulitis may indicate a deeper placed infection such as soft tissue abscess or osteomyelitis.

Group A streptococci and staphylococci are the most common pathogens, but the causative organism may vary considerably.

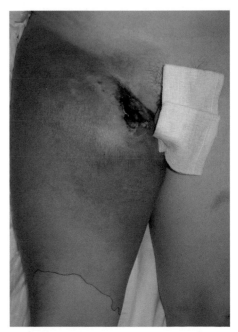

Figure 10.1 Spreading cellulitis of the right groin resulting from a vascular access device. Image supplied by Mr H. S. Khaira, Heart of England Foundation Trust.

Diagnosis

Blood cultures should be taken. There is little merit in skin biopsy and culture as the inevitable mixed growth is unlikely to be helpful. Swabs of areas with frank pus may provide positive cultures. Imaging of deeper structures should be carried out if the history and examination suggest deep infection.

Treatment

High-dose flucloxacillin will cover most staphylococci and streptococci. If there is a possibility of MRSA infection then vancomycin should be added. In many areas with outpatient-based antibiotic regimes, ceftriaxone is used for ease of administration (once daily IV). IV antibiotics should continue until there is improvement in systemic features. If improvement is not seen, further assessment and debridement of necrotic areas may be required.

Special cases

Circumferential cellulitis

If the affected area completely surrounds a limb or trunk, there is a danger of progression to full thickness necrosis. This needs very close observation and surgical debridement may be needed.

Cellulitis of hands and forearms

The fascial compartments in these areas are tight, and oedema can rapidly cause a compartment syndrome. If there is pain or limitation of movement of wrist or fingers, urgent surgical review must be requested.

Periorbital cellulitis

Whilst causes and risk factors are similar, the possibility of orbital and sinus involvement requires more detailed initial investigations including computerized tomography (CT) scan and involvement of specialist teams. Cavernous sinus thrombosis can be an underlying cause and magnetic resonance imaging (MRI) is the investigation of choice if this is suspected. Symptoms include headache, nausea and vomiting.

Perineal cellulitis

Fornier's gangrene is a polymicrobial infection of the perineal area with necrosis and rapid spread along fascial planes. This is an emergency situation and surgery is urgently required.

Necrotizing fasciitis

This is covered in greater detail in Chapter 11. It is a rapidly progressing severe infection that spreads along fascial planes leading to local neurovascular damage, ischemia and necrosis. There is a significant systemic reaction leading to sepsis and progressing to septic shock and its consequences. Surgical debridement is almost always necessary and the patient will need to be managed in a high dependency setting. Seek senior and expert help immediately.

Osteomyelitis

This is a destructive inflammation of the bone cortex (Figure 10.2), with sequestrum formation that can cause surrounding bone ischaemia leading to poor antibiotic penetration. The chronic phase of osteomyelitis may present with pain, fracture, systemic upset or overlying cellulitis. Treatment is difficult and protracted. Expert advice must be sought from orthopaedic surgeons and bone infection specialists.

Bone aspiration or biopsy sent for culture will guide therapy but treatment should certainly cover staphylococci, for example, with high-dose flucloxacillin and gentamicin. Due to the poor penetration of antibiotics associated with this condition, courses of some weeks are frequently used.

Pneumonia

Pneumonia (Figure 10.3) can be caused by bacteria, viruses or by atypical agents including fungi. Pneumonia classically presents with a productive cough, purulent sputum, fever and systemic illness.

The causative organisms vary greatly and likely pathogens will be determined by history and examination. In broad terms, it is possible to separate out pneumonias into community or hospital acquired. Whilst *Streptococcus pneumoniae* remains the

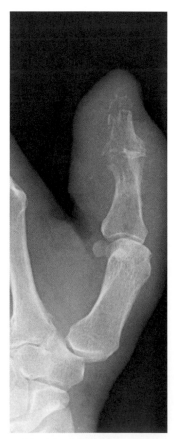

Figure 10.2 Osteomyelitis of the thumb, with bony destruction.

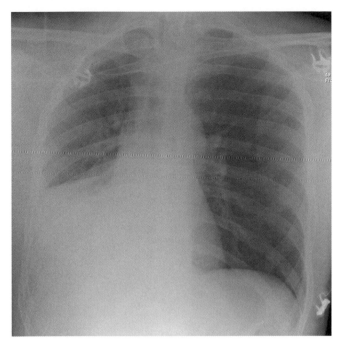

Figure 10.3 Chest radiograph of a right lower lobe pneumonia with collapse, loss of lung volume manifest as a shift of the mediastinum to the right.

most common agent whether in the community or in hospitals, there is an increased risk of enterobacteria and pseudomonas in institutionalized patients and these must be considered. Patients who have undergone invasive ventilation may develop ventilator-associated pneumonia. Intensive care units have developed care bundles to reduce the incidence of this condition, which is sometimes associated with subclinical aspiration of gastric contents.

It should be remembered that, despite media attention to resistant organisms, the pneumococcus remains one of the most virulent organisms once a bacteraemia develops and can produce a fulminant and rapidly fatal illness (<24 hours) in susceptible individuals.

Diagnosis

The British Thoracic Society guidelines recommend that all patients admitted from the community with pneumonia be assessed using the CURB (or CURB-65) score, which has been validated to stratify risk of death and can be used as a marker of severity. A CURB-65 of >3 mandates admission to an acute unit (Box 10.2).

Box 10.2 **The CURB score**

- Confusion or altered mental state
- Urea: raised >7 mmol/l
- Respiratory rate: raised >30/minute
- Blood pressure (BP): (systolic <90 mmHg and/or diastolic <60 mmHg)

Patients with two or more of these and aged above 65 (corresponding to a CURB-65 score of over 3) have a high risk of death and should be managed aggressively in hospital. For other cases, the patient may still require hospital care depending on other factors such as co-morbidities. A patient with a score of zero may be managed in the community.

A chest X-ray may demonstrate areas of lung affected and associated effusions or structural abnormalities. Effusions provide the opportunity for diagnostic and therapeutic aspiration. Those with clinical and radiological signs of consolidation may benefit from bronchoscopy, particularly if an underlying lesion is suspected. The sample should be sent for pH, protein, lactate dehydrogenase (LDH), glucose, microscopy and culture. As a rule of thumb, if the glucose is low and protein is high, or if the pH is low, the fluid is likely to be an empyema. If the fluid is infected, the empyema must be removed using a large-gauge chest drain.

Arterial blood gases will help assess the severity of pneumonia and the level of oxygen therapy required. Blood cultures should be taken. If purulent sputum can be collected, it should be analysed with the results interpreted in context.

Treatment

First-line antibiotic choice depends on previous history of antibiotic exposure and local microbiology guidelines. An example of such a guideline is given in Box 10.3. Patients with recurrent infections or with underlying bronchiectasis should have a careful review of previously isolated organisms. Severe chest infections in young adults should prompt consideration of an occult immunocompromised state. In the first instance, history and basic investigations should be reviewed but human immunodeficiency virus (HIV) may need to be considered.

Box 10.3 **Example of antibiotic guidelines for pneumonia*,†**

Community-acquired pneumonia
(evidence of consolidation on chest X-ray; document CURB-65 score)

Mild – Moderate
Amoxicillin 500 mg tds orally and clarithromycin* 500 mg bd orally
Penicillin allergy: clarithromycin 500 mg bd orally

Severe
(that is, 3 or more of CURB-65: confusion, urea >7, respiratory rate (RR) >30, diastolic BP <60, age >65 years)
Benzylpenicillin 1.2 g qds IV and clarithromycin 500 mg bd IV
Penicillin allergy: levofloxacin 500 mg bd IV and clarithromycin 500 mg bd IV
Review at 48-hourly intervals, change to oral amoxicillin and clarithromycin once improving and able to tolerate oral diet

Critically ill (requiring Critical Care admission or review)
Levofloxacin 500 mg bd IV and benzylpenicillin 1.2 g qds IV
Penicillin allergy: levofloxacin 500 mg bd IV and clarithromycin 500 mg bd IV)

If urinary sepsis is also likely, consider adding gentamicin
160 mg stat IV

Infective exacerbation of chronic obstructive pulmonary disease (COPD) (with purulent sputum)

Doxycycline 200 mg stat, then 100 mg od orally
OR
Amoxicillin 500 mg tds orally
For type II respiratory failure: seek respiratory team advice,
amoxicillin 1 g tds IV

---

*Apply Severe Sepsis Screening Tool for all cases of pneumonia.
†All antibiotic prescriptions must be reviewed at 48 hours, or sooner if culture and sensitivity results are available.
Adapted with permission from Heart of England NHS Foundation Trust, February 2007.

In the immunocompromised patient, particularly if the features are anything other than classical, viral and fungal infections should be considered and covered (Chapter 12). Recurrent infections may indicate an endobronchial lesion, and a thorough evaluation must be made to exclude malignancy.

Special cases

Patients with structural lung disease or chronic obstructive pulmonary disease (COPD)

These patients are more susceptible to infections. There is some evidence that patients with exacerbations of chronic obstructive pulmonary disease (COPD) and altered coloured sputum should be treated empirically with antibiotics (doxycycline is acceptable).

Aspiration pneumonia

Inhalation of gastric or oropharyngeal contents causes chemical pneumonitis; this inflammation restricts clearance of airway secretions and may lead to pneumonia. Chemical pneumonitis will not respond to antibiotics, and antibiotic treatment is best limited to patients who mount a systemic response (indicating superadded infection). Most patients in the community who aspirate will have normal upper airway flora made up principally of *S. pneumoniae*, *S. aureus*, *Haemophilus* and β-haemolytic streptococci. However, in hospitalized or recently discharged patients, previous antibiotic use and exposure may have changed the flora and whilst streptococcal species still predominate, there will be increased frequencies of Enterobacteriaciae (*Klebsiella pneumoniae*, *Escherichia coli*, *Enterobacter* spp.), *Pseudomonas aeruginosa* and anaerobic species.

Because of the wide range of possible pathogens, the antibiotics chosen in aspiration pneumonia should initially be broad spectrum and be capable of penetrating into lung parenchyma in high concentrations.

Line-related sepsis

Central lines, peripheral cannulae and other intravascular catheters can all become colonized and infected. Causes are poor technique at insertion, poor ongoing care and seeding onto lines from a bacteraemia. Patients may present with florid bacteraemia with only minor skin changes around the catheter insertion site. The true incidence of this remains unclear but up to 50% of healthcare-associated infections (HCAIs) have been attributed to invasive lines. Bacteraemia is estimated to complicate 0.3–1% of peripheral and 8% of central venous lines. Infection prevention related to line placement is discussed in Chapter 8.

Causative organisms are listed in Box 10.4.

Box 10.4 **Causative organisms for line sepsis**

Coagulase negative staphylococci	35%
Staphylococcus aureus including MRSA	25%
Enterobacteria	
Klebsiella	
Pseudomonas	
Entercocci	
Streptococci	
Candida spp	

Diagnosis

If a central line is thought culpable, paired blood cultures should be taken from it and a peripheral site. The entry puncture point should also be swabbed if it looks inflamed or if there is frank pus. Peripheral lines are also commonly associated with hospital-acquired bacteraemias and close monitoring of surrounding phlebitis and cannula patency should be maintained, for example, using the Visual Infusion Phlebitis (VIP) Score (Figure 10.4). Hospitals are now using care bundles for peripheral line insertion and ongoing care, with many mandating that a peripheral venous cannula should remain in situ for no longer than 72 hours.

Treatment

Treatment requires the line to be removed as soon as possible. Antibiotics should cover staphylococci empirically, for example, using high-dose flucloxacillin. Microbiology services should be consulted as early as possible. Infected lines should only be removed once satisfactory alternative access is available, but time is of the essence.

Meningitis

Meningitis is an inflammatory condition affecting the meninges of the brain. Bacterial, viral, parasitic, infiltrative, metabolic and immune-mediated forms of meningitis occur.

It is often difficult to distinguish between the causes of meningitis on clinical criteria alone, especially in sick patients, and so a high index of suspicion for bacterial meningitis is sensible in view of its immediately life-threatening nature.

Clinical features

Headache (87% of cases), neck stiffness (83%) and fever are the most common presenting features. Their collective absence makes

Phlebitis Score

All patients with an intravenous (IV) access device should have the IV site checked every shift for signs of infusion phlebitis. The subsequent score and action(s) taken (if any) must be documented on the cannula record form.

The cannula site must also be observed:
• When bolus injections are administered
• IV flow rates are checked or altered
• When solution containers are changed

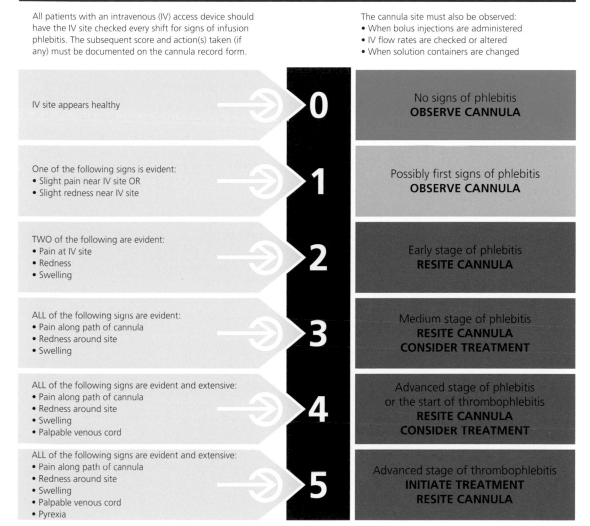

IV site appears healthy

0 No signs of phlebitis
OBSERVE CANNULA

One of the following signs is evident:
• Slight pain near IV site OR
• Slight redness near IV site

1 Possibly first signs of phlebitis
OBSERVE CANNULA

TWO of the following are evident:
• Pain at IV site
• Redness
• Swelling

2 Early stage of phlebitis
RESITE CANNULA

ALL of the following signs are evident:
• Pain along path of cannula
• Redness around site
• Swelling

3 Medium stage of phlebitis
RESITE CANNULA
CONSIDER TREATMENT

ALL of the following signs are evident and extensive:
• Pain along path of cannula
• Redness around site
• Swelling
• Palpable venous cord

4 Advanced stage of phlebitis or the start of thrombophlebitis
RESITE CANNULA
CONSIDER TREATMENT

ALL of the following signs are evident and extensive:
• Pain along path of cannula
• Redness around site
• Swelling
• Palpable venous cord
• Pyrexia

5 Advanced stage of thrombophlebitis
INITIATE TREATMENT
RESITE CANNULA

Figure 10.4 Visual Infusion Phlebitis (VIP) Score. With permission from Andrew Jackson – Consultant Nurse, Intravenous Therapy & Care, The Rotherham NHS Foundation Trust. (Adapted from Jackson, 1998.)

meningitis very unlikely. In addition, other signs of meningeal irritation may be seen – photophobia, irritability and delirium. In some, seizures are seen. Kernig's sign (with hips and knees flexed, extending the knees beyond 135 degrees causes pain in the supine patient) is often quoted as being diagnostic but cannot be relied upon to include or exclude a diagnosis. The rapidly spreading petechial rash, typical of meningococcaemia (*Neisseria meningitidis*), can occur with or without meningitis, and may precede other symptoms by up to a day. Similarly, meningococcal meningitis can occur in the absence of a rash.

The typical rash of purpura fulminans is seen in Figure 10.5.

Incidence

Vaccination programmes (predominantly pneumovax and haemophilus influenzae type b (HiB)) have reduced the incidence of pneumococcal meningitis, but it remains high and tends to occur

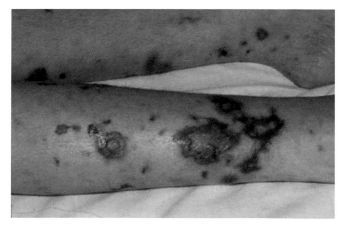

Figure 10.5 The typical rash of meningococcal septicaemia, caused by *Neisseria meningitidis*. With permission from the Wellcome Trust Photographic Library.

in clusters in areas of close contact and high density such as university halls of residence and schools.

Causative organisms are listed in Box 10.5.

Box 10.5 **Causative organisms for meningitis (most common first)**

Neisseria meningitidis	Gram-negative diplococcus
	Vaccines for serogoups A, C but not B
Streptococcus pneumoniae	Commensal from oropharynx
	Especially following trauma/ neurosurgery
Haemophilus influenzae type B	Increasingly rare due to introduction of HiB vaccine
Listeria monocytogenes	Old, very young, immunosuppressed, alcoholics
Mycobacterium tuberculosis	Less common but should be considered in high-risk patients

Diagnosis

Lumbar puncture (LP) should ideally be performed before antibiotics are given, but should not delay their administration. LP findings are listed in Box 10.6.

Box 10.6 **Findings on lumbar puncture**

Type	Glucose	Protein	Cell type
Acute bacterial meningitis	Low	High	Polymorphonuclear cells >300/mm^3
Acute viral meningitis	Normal	Normal or high	Mononuclear cells <300/mm^3
Tuberculous meningitis	Low	High	Pleocytosis, mixed <300/mm^3
Fungal meningitis	Low	High	<300/mm^3
Malignant meningitis	Low	High	Mononucleacytes
Subarachnoid haemorrhage	Normal	Normal or high	Erythrocytes and xanthochromia

CT imaging is not essential if there is no focal neurology or altered mental state. A CT scan cannot completely exclude structural problems or raised intracranial pressure, and treatment should certainly not be delayed for such imaging to occur.

Peripheral blood cultures should be taken and a sample retained for polymerase chain reaction (PCR) to look for DNA traces of bacteria and viruses; this is particularly useful if prior antibiotic administration has caused the cerebrospinal fluid (CSF) to be sterile.

Testing for toxoplasmosis, Epstein-Barr virus, cytomegalovirus and fungal infection may be relevant in some immunocompromised states.

Treatment

It is widely recommended that 2 g of IV ceftriaxone with 8–12 mg of dexamethasone be given as soon as possible. Ampicillin should be added if *Listeria* is suspected. If there is an indolent history and suggestion of altered behaviour, viral meningitis and encephalitis must be considered, and acyclovir should be added.

The use of early steroids has been demonstrated to improve outcome by reducing the inflammatory cascade seen during acute bacterial cell killing with first-dose antibiotics. This is especially the case in pneumococcal disease.

Do not delay antibiotics whilst getting CT imaging or an LP.

Ten days of IV antibiotic therapy is normally recommended for bacterial meningitis, narrowed to the causative organism once known.

Close 'kissing' contacts should be offered prophylaxis and public health teams should be informed in most countries.

Special cases

Tuberculous meningitis

Tuberculous (TB) meningitis should be considered in the differential diagnoses of patients from high-risk groups, typically presenting with a subacute/chronic picture with patients having variable pyrexia, malaise, headaches and lymphadenopathy. Cranial nerve deficits may be seen and there may be a raised intracranial pressure.

TB meningitis can be staged according to the degree of neurological impairment (Box 10.7).

Box 10.7 **Staging of tuberculous meningitis**

Stage 1	No change in mental function, no deficits, no hydrocephalus
Stage 2	Confusion and/or evidence of neurologic deficit
Stage 3	Stupor and lethargy

Encephalitis

Encephalitis (inflammation of brain tissue) often has a slowly progressing course with myalgia and mild features of meningism. Encephalitis caused by herpes viruses can present with a rash and lymphadenopathy.

Most commonly there is a behavioural change with altered personality and diffuse neurological deficits. Confusion, coma and death can occur rapidly.

Suspected encephalitis should be treated urgently with acyclovir. It is used in herpes simplex virus (HSV) and varicella zoster virus (VZV) disease to reduce the clinical duration and severity. In HIV patients, HSV may be acyclovir resistant and foscarnet should be substituted. Generally, co-treatment for bacterial meningitis should be started, as it is often very difficult to distinguish the clinical features. LP and blood culture are still indicated, and once results are known, therapy can be rationalized.

Endocarditis

Infective endocarditis (IE) can present with features of a multisystem disorder in an acute, subacute or chronic manner. Bacteraemia, anaemia, septic embolization, immune-mediated phenomena and valvular decay with a compromised circulation may all be present. Diagnosis is often difficult and treatment can be prolonged. Previously damaged, prosthetic or congenitally abnormal valves are more susceptible, though the incidence of endocarditis in normal native valves is also high.

Group B haemolytic streptococci are most commonly responsible but staphylococci, mycobacteria and enterococci are all found. Fungal infections are much less common and usually confined to the immunosuppressed.

In patients with a history of IV drug abuse, right-sided endocarditis (principally tricuspid valve) is more likely, with *S. aureus* being the most common pathogen.

Aortic valve endocarditis is associated with local abscess formation, which can lead to complete collapse of valve integrity. It is often heralded by a lengthening PR interval on an electrocardiogram (ECG).

Endocarditis can also occur with infection in an indwelling vascular line or pacing wire.

Diagnosis is made using the Dukes University criteria (Box 10.8).

Box 10.8 **Diagnostic criteria for infective endocarditis (Dukes University)**

Two major criteria, or one major and three minor criteria, or five minor criteria

Major criteria

A. Positive blood culture for infective endocarditis (IE), defined as one of the following:

- Typical micro-organism consistent with IE from two separate blood cultures, as noted below:

  Viridans group streptococci, *Streptococcus bovis*, or HACEK (**H**aemophilus, **A**ctinobacillus actinomycetemcomitans, **C**ardiobacterium hominis, **E**ikenella corrodens, **K**ingella) group, or
  Community-acquired *S. aureus* or enterococci, in the absence of a primary focus

- Microorganisms consistent with IE from persistently positive blood cultures defined as follows:

  Two positive cultures of blood samples drawn >12 hours apart, or All of three or a majority of four separate cultures of blood (with first and last samples drawn 1 hour apart)

B. Evidence of endocardial involvement

  Positive echocardiogram for IE demonstrating vegetations
  New valvular regurgitation (worsening or changing of pre-existing murmur not sufficient)

Minor criteria

- Predisposition: predisposing heart condition or intravenous drug use
- Fever: temperature >38.0°C
- Vascular phenomena: major arterial emboli, septic pulmonary infarcts, mycotic aneurysm, intracranial haemorrhage, conjunctival haemorrhages and Janeway lesions
- Immunologic phenomena: glomerulonephritis, Osler's nodes, Roth spots, and rheumatoid factor

---

- Microbiological evidence: positive blood culture but does not meet a major criterion as noted above or serological evidence of active infection with organism consistent with IE
- Echocardiographic findings: consistent with IE but do not meet a major criterion as noted above

A transthoracic ECG will not exclude a diagnosis of endocarditis. A transoesphageal ECG is more sensitive (around 90%) in detecting vegetations and perivalvular abscesses. A high clinical suspicion must be acted upon even if imaging is not supportive.

Treatment

If organisms are yet to be identified and the patient is unwell, treatment should be started immediately. Streptococcal and staphylococcal species remain the most common and so high-dose IV broad-spectrum penicillin or cephalosporin, with gentamicin, can be started. However, in injecting drug users or those with prostheses, there is a possibility of methicillin-resistant staphylococcus and so vancomycin becomes first-line empirical therapy (Box 10.9).

Box 10.9 **Antimicrobial treatment if therapy is urgent and the causative organism unidentified**

Native valves	
Vancomycin 15 mg/kg IV every 12 hours	4–6 weeks
+ gentamicin 1.0 mg/kg IV every 8 hours	2 weeks
Prosthetic valves	
Vancomycin 15 mg/kg IV every 12 hours	4–6 weeks
+ rifampicin 300–450 mg PO every 8 hours	4–6 weeks
+ gentamicin 1.0 mg/kg IV every 8 hours	2 weeks

Sources of ongoing bacteraemia such as poor dentition, indwelling lines and abscesses must be sought and excluded or controlled. Once a likely pathogen has been identified, microbiology should be consulted on the most appropriate antibiotics to be used.

If there is heart failure or any cardiac rhythm abnormality, cardiology advice should be sought immediately. In cases of severe valvular destruction, surgery may be required.

Diarrhoeal illnesses

These are very common. In susceptible patients, *C. difficile* must be suspected, but most commonly the episode is virally mediated and self-limiting. *C. difficile* infection is covered in Chapter 11.

Conclusion

This has been, by necessity, a brief overview. What will be apparent is that infections manifest in a syndrome-like manner and the finding of sepsis tend to be common. It is vitally important to look hard for the source and consider confounding elements when planning treatment. Use of antibiotics must be pragmatic, early and then focused once further information is available. Antibiotics, however, are not adequate by themselves; nutrition, hydration, mobility, thromboembolic prophylaxis and intercurrent health problems must all be considered.

Further reading and resources

British Thoracic Society Pneumonia Guidelines Committee. BTS Guidelines for the Management of Community Acquired Pneumonia in Adults, 2004 update. Accessible from www.brit-thoracic.org.uk.

    The British Thoracic Society has regular updates for the management of community- and hospital-acquired pneumonia. It also has the current recommendations for tuberculosis (TB). It provides a good resource to help understand how such guidelines are made and why.

Elliott TE, Worthington T, Osman H & Gill M, eds. *Medical Microbiology and Infection*, 4th edn. Blackwell Publishing Ltd, Oxford, 2007.

    An excellent view of applied microbiology with useful advice on how to apply a systematic approach to the management of infections whilst giving lots of basic science information to underpin practice.

Health Protection Agency website www.hpa.org.uk. This is the main portal of the Health Protection Agency and it has lots of useful information and links to background reading covering a wealth of conditions. The hospital-acquired infections (HAI) resource is particularly relevant and will empower doctors and nurses of all grades to understand how to avoid and manage such problems.

CHAPTER 11

Presentations in Surgical Patients

Jonathan Stewart and Sian Abbott

Good Hope Hospital, Heart of England NHS Foundation Trust, Birmingham, UK

OVERVIEW

- Surgical patients with sepsis do not always present with textbook signs and symptoms
- If a patient unexpectedly deteriorates following a bowel resection, an anastamotic leak must be considered
- The principles of treatment are to drain collections, treat the disease process and provide adequate supportive measures

Identification

Sepsis may present to the surgeon as a result of three main processes:

1 As a consequence of a disease process
   for example, acute diverticulitis, perforated duodenal ulcer.
2 As a direct complication of surgery
   for example, anastomotic leak, unrecognized bowel injury during surgery.
3 As a complication relating to iatrogenic insult
   for example, nosocomial infections, catheter and line sepsis.

This chapter will focus on sepsis arising from intra-abdominal pathology. Perhaps the symptom most specific to the surgical team is that of abdominal pain. This can occur as a presenting symptom or as a new or worsening sign post-operatively. Peritonitis is a clinical diagnosis. Pain is the most common symptom, which may be diffuse or localized and is usually constant. Anorexia, malaise, nausea and vomiting are common. On examination, the patient will lie still with shallow respiration. Palpation of the abdomen exacerbates the pain and may well demonstrate tenderness, guarding and rebound tenderness. The site of maximum tenderness is often the site of pathology. The Mannheim Peritonitis Index (Table 11.1) is an objective scoring system for predicting outcome in patients with peritonitis.

Post-operative peritonitis occurs in 1–20% of patients undergoing laparotomy. Post-operative patients may be difficult to assess as wound tenderness, analgesia and antibiotics may confuse new symptoms and signs.

In the elderly population, clinical presentation may reflect the organ system most vulnerable to the systemic inflammatory process or disturbances in blood flow, for example, the central nervous system (CNS), rather than the organ that is diseased. The elderly patient with sepsis may present with agitation, lethargy or following a fall. Localization of pain may not be reliable, and fever may be less marked.

Assessing an unstable patient on Critical Care for signs of abdominal sepsis requiring intervention is often difficult. Sedation, paralysis, mechanical ventilation and antibiotics may mask signs. A new complication may have developed, or there may be ongoing sepsis in a patient with recent faecal peritonitis. Missed abdominal sepsis in a patient with organ failure is almost always fatal. A gradual deterioration with no obvious cause, an increasing requirement for inotropes or vasopressors, or the gradual onset of renal failure may be the only signs. Where there is diagnostic doubt in a patient with progressive sepsis a second look – laparotomy or computerized tomography (CT) imaging (if the patient is stable for transfer) may be required.

Table 11.1 The Mannheim Peritonitis Index: risk factors, scores and mortality.

Mannheim Peritonitis Index			
Risk Factor	**Weight**	**Score**	**Mortality**
Age >50 yr	5	<21	0–2.3%
Female	5		
Organ failure*	7	21–29	60–65%
Malignancy	4		
Pre-operative duration of peritonitis >24 h	4	>29	80–100%
Origin of sepsis not colonic	4		
Diffuse generalized peritonitis	6		
Exudates			
Clear	0		
Cloudy	6		
Faecal	12		

*Organ Failure
Kidney: creatinine >177 μmol/l, urea >167 mmol/l, oliguria <20 ml/h
Lung: PaO_2 <50 mmHg, $PaCO_2$ >50 mmHg
Shock: hypodynamic, hyperdynamic
Intestinal: obstruction, paralysis >24 h or complete mechanical ileus.

ABC of Sepsis. Edited by Ron Daniels and Tim Nutbeam. © 2010 by Blackwell Publishing, ISBN: 978-1-4501-8194-5.

Aetiology

Wound infections

The principle source of infection in surgical wounds is the patient's own (commensal) bacterial flora. Infection rates relate to the classification of wound and type of surgery (Table 11.2). Diagnosis is based on clinical findings with local signs such as erythema, induration, warmth and purulent discharge (Figure 11.1). Systemic signs may also be present. Infected wounds should be opened, fluid collections allowed to drain and bacterial cultures from pus obtained. An infected wound will rarely respond to antibiotics alone.

Perforated viscus

The common sites of perforation are the duodenum (peptic ulcer), the sigmoid colon (diverticulitis) and the appendix (acute appendicitis). Small bowel perforations may occur secondary to obstruction, ischaemia and Crohn's disease. An erect chest radiograph may show free gas under the diaphragm, confirming perforation (Figure 11.2). A small diverticular perforation may cause localized

Table 11.2 Surgical wound classification and infection rates.

Classification	Infection rate (%)	Definition
Clean	<2	Incision through non-inflamed tissue. Not entering a hollow viscus
Clean-contaminated	10	Incision through a hollow viscus other than colon, with minimal contamination
Contaminated	20	Incision through a hollow viscus with gross spillage or incision through colon. Human/animal bite. Open fracture
Dirty	40	Faecal peritonitis, traumatic wound contaminated for >4 h, frank pus

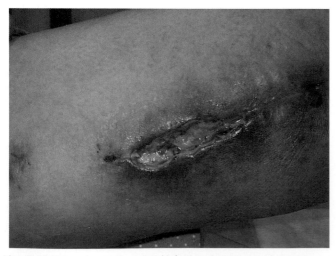

Figure 11.1 A post-operative wound infection. Courtesy Mr Harmeet S Khaira FRCS.

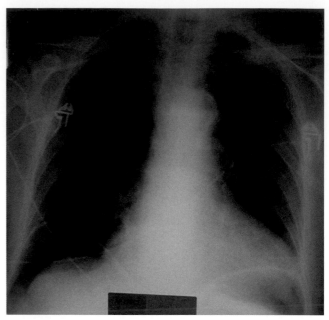

Figure 11.2 An erect chest radiograph showing free gas under the diaphragm. Courtesy Mr Harmeet S Khaira FRCS.

peritonitis or abscess formation. However, a large perforation causes sudden overwhelming faecal peritonitis with septic shock. This requires urgent fluid resuscitation, involvement of Critical Care and emergency laparotomy.

Anastomotic leak

In patients who have undergone bowel resection, a slow recovery or unexpected deterioration following surgery should raise the suspicion of an anastomotic leak. These classically present between days 5 and 7. Patients often present with subtle, non-specific signs such as arrhythmias. Extravasation of fluid laden with bacteria leads to local abscess formation, fistula, anastomotic breakdown, wound dehiscence and localized or generalized peritonitis. Risk factors for anastomotic dehiscence are listed in Table 11.3.

A high index of suspicion on the part of the surgical team is required when patients fail to make progress or clinically deteriorate. Diagnosis may include imaging of the anastomosis with a water-soluble contrast enema or a CT scan.

A small, contained leak in a stable patient may be managed conservatively. Reoperation is indicated in an uncontrolled leak. This may require defunctioning of the bowel by means of a stoma and drainage of the sepsis.

Table 11.3 Factors associated with anastamotic leaks.

Poor technique	Tension, poor blood supply, unrecognized mesenteric vessel damage, poor suture technique
Local factors	Distal obstruction, ischaemia, ongoing peritonitis, gross bowel wall oedema
Systemic factors	Hypovolaemic shock, age, malnutrition, immunosuppression

Table 11.4 Symptoms, signs and aetiology of abdominal abscesses.

Anatomical space	Cause	Symptoms	Signs
Subphrenic			
Left	Post-operative complication of surgery to stomach, tail of pancreas, spleen and splenic flexure of colon	Hiccups, shoulder tip pain, anorexia, abdominal or chest pain	Swinging pyrexia, abdominal tenderness, collapse of lung base and pleural effusion
Right	Perforating cholecystitis, perforated duodenal ulcer, duodenal stump leak following gastric surgery		
Subhepatic	Cholecystitis, appendicitis, perforated duodenal ulcer and following upper abdominal surgery	As above	As above
Lesser sac	Infected pseudocyst following acute severe pancreatitis	Early satiety, malaise, abdominal pain	Swinging pyrexia, palpable mass
Pelvis	Appendicitis, pelvic inflammatory disease, anastamotic leak, diverticulitis and following rectal surgery	Diarrhoea, passing mucus per rectum, tenesmus, frequency of micturition	Abdominal/pelvic tenderness, palpable mass on rectal examination
Inter-loop	Post-operative complication of generalized peritonitis	Malaise, anorexia	Failure to progress

Abscesses

Intra-abdominal abscesses are localized collections of pus that are confined in the peritoneal cavity by an inflammatory barrier. This barrier may include the omentum, inflammatory adhesions or contiguous viscera. The abscesses usually contain a mixture of aerobic and anaerobic bacteria from the gastrointestinal (GI) tract.

The development of an intra-abdominal abscess is determined by local conditions, the nature of the disease and the patient's response to it. The distribution is directly related to the precipitating lesion and to the potential peritoneal spaces (Table 11.4).

The presentation of such an abscess may be variable. The only indication may be a prolonged ileus, mild liver dysfunction or intermittent polymicrobial bacteraemia.

Figure 11.3 shows a large pelvic abscess.

The kidneys, pancreas, psoas muscles and major vessels reside in the retroperitoneal space. A psoas abscess may develop following spread of infection from the kidneys, pancreas, appendix, colon and vertebral bodies. Patients may present acutely with pyrexia, malaise, weight loss and pain, which may be referred to the hip, groin or knee. There may be concurrent chronic illnesses such as diabetes mellitus, Crohn's disease or malignancies. Tuberculosis of the spine is an important cause of retroperitoneal abscess in the immunocompromised patient. A plain abdominal radiograph may show loss of psoas margins and ultrasound/CT scan is usually diagnostic. Management depends on the underlying cause but involves drainage of the sepsis and treatment of the underlying pathology.

Septic arthritis

Septic arthritis, the infection of one or more joints, is usually bacterial in origin. Common causative organisms are *Staphylococcus aureus, Haemophilus influenzae, Neisseria gonorrhoea* and *Escherichia coli*. It presents with pain, swelling, fever and reduced movement and is a surgical emergency as delays in treatment lead to destruction of the articular cartilage by bacterial proteolytic enzymes. Where there is a joint prosthesis, the onset is usually more insidious, with gradually increasing pain, sinus formation and loosening of the prosthesis. Diagnosis is by aspiration, Gram stain and culture of fluid from the joint. Plain film findings of septic arthritis include joint effusion, soft tissue swelling, periarticular osteoporosis, loss of joint space, marginal and central erosions and bone ankylosis. Treatment involves intravenous antibiotics, analgesia and open or arthroscopic aspiration and washout of the joint.

Diabetic foot

About 15% of people with diabetes mellitus develop foot ulceration, which is complicated by osteomyelitis in two-thirds of cases. Factors associated with infection are duration of diabetes mellitus (>10 years), peripheral neuropathy, peripheral vascular disease, poor glycaemic control and disruption of skin integrity (for example, penetrating injury, fungal infection). Presentation may be delayed as the ulcers are often painless secondary to diabetic neuropathy. Erythema, swelling, ulceration and purulent discharge may be present. Limb-threatening infections are associated with polymicrobial infection, deep-seated abscess, advancing cellulitis, gangrene and osteomyelitis. Plain X-ray is useful but the changes of osteomyelitis are often not present for up to 3 weeks after the bone is infected. Debridement should include removal of all dead

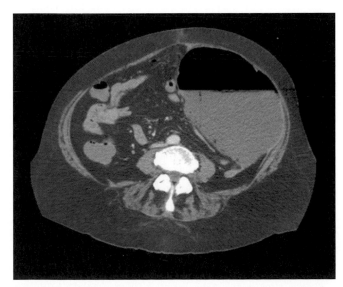

Figure 11.3 A computerized tomographic (CT) image of a large diverticular abscess, with a gas – fluid level. Courtesy Dr Morgan S Cleasby.

and necrotic tissue including infected bone, with maintenance of functional integrity of the foot as the goal. Prevention, crucial to reducing the risk of an injury that can lead to ulcer formation, involves patient education regarding foot hygiene, nail care and proper footwear.

Necrotizing fasciitis

Necrotizing fasciitis is a soft tissue infection, characterized by rapidly progressing necrosis of the subcutaneous tissue and fascia with relative sparing of the skin and muscle. The area becomes tender, swollen and erythematous (Figure 11.4). Pain is often more severe than the visible signs would suggest. There may be signs of sepsis. Most cases are polymicrobial in origin; however, approximately 10% of cases are monomicrobial infections with group A streptococci, which can produce pyrogenic exotoxins (bacterial products directly causing inflammation and fever). A CT scan may demonstrate fat stranding and gas tracking along fascial planes (Figure 11.5). Definitive treatment is surgical and delay is associated with an increase in mortality. Early debridement to normal healthy tissue is essential and may need to be extensive. Broad-spectrum intravenous antibiotics and supportive care in a high dependency unit are required, with a likely need for repeat debridements.

Severe acute pancreatitis

Severe acute pancreatitis is an inflammatory condition involving pancreatic acinar cells. The result is the development of a systemic inflammatory response syndrome (SIRS). The clinical picture mirrors that of severe sepsis, and may lead to multiple organ dysfunction. Septic complications of pancreatitis may occur, but are rare, and include infected pseudocyst and infected pancreatic necrosis. A pseudocyst is a collection of pancreatic fluid within a wall of granulation tissue, which usually requires at least 4 weeks to form. This fluid can become infected, forming an abscess. Treatment is drainage, either by percutaneous, transgastric or surgical means. Pancreatic necrosis may be focal or diffuse,

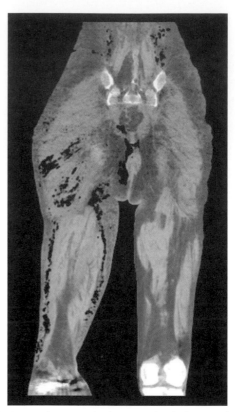

Figure 11.5 A coronal computerized tomographic (CT) image of a patient with necrotizing fasciitis. Gas can be seen in the subcutaneous tissues. Courtesy Dr Morgan J Cleasby.

and infected pancreatic necrosis is a life-threatening complication. Diagnosis is made with CT-guided aspiration of necrotic tissue and a positive microbiological culture. These may be managed conservatively with percutaneous drainage but occasionally laparotomy with debridement of all necrotic tissue may be required.

Acute cholecystitis

Acute cholecystitis usually presents with right upper quadrant pain and signs of sepsis. Diagnosis is confirmed by ultrasound scan, showing a thick-walled gallbladder with stones. An empyema (abscess of the gallbladder) may develop. Gallbladder necrosis may occur leading to perforation and either localized or generalized peritonitis.

Acalculous cholecystitis (that is, in the absence of stones) usually occurs during the course of a prolonged critical illness. Ultrasound or CT may confirm the diagnosis with pericholecystic fluid or intramural gas. Management includes cholecystectomy (open or laparoscopic) or transhepatic, percutaneous cholecystostomy if the patient is not fit for surgery.

Acute emphysematous cholecystitis is caused by polymicrobial infection with gas-forming organisms (*E. coli*, *Clostridium welchii*, streptococci). It occurs predominantly in males with diabetes.

Clostridium difficile colitis

Clostridium difficile is an anaerobic, gram-positive spore-forming bacillus that produces two toxins, A and B. A is directly cytotoxic

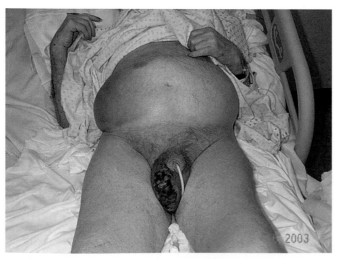

Figure 11.4 Necrotizing fasciitis of the scrotum (Fournier's gangrene) spreading to the abdominal wall and right flank. Courtesy Mr Harmeet S Khaira FRCS.

and causes an inflammatory infiltration of the colonic mucosa which then becomes necrotic. Approximately 2% of the healthy population carry the organism. It is spread by the faecal – oral route, and indirectly through spores on surfaces. *C. difficile* can cause antibiotic-associated diarrhoea and pseudomembranous colitis, a more serious condition. Toxic megacolon is a life-threatening complication of colitis, characterized by acute dilatation of all or part of the colon and signs of sepsis. Surgery is indicated for colonic perforation, peritonitis, fulminant colitis not responding to medical therapy and toxic megacolon. The usual procedure is subtotal colectomy and ileostomy.

The mortality from *C. difficile* colitis currently stands at 6–30%. In the United Kingdom, *C. difficile* has contributed to approximately 3000–4000 deaths per annum over the last few years.

Management

Management of the surgical patient with sepsis requires a multidisciplinary approach including surgeons, intensivists and anaesthetists, radiologists, microbiologists and nutrition support teams. Key stages include drainage of collections, debridement of devitalized tissue, removal of infected foreign bodies, definitive measures to correct the pathology and supportive treatment for failing organ systems.

Conservative

Certain conditions causing localized sepsis such as an appendix mass or acute diverticulitis may be managed with medical therapy. Patients require close observation and regular assessment. If they fail to improve or deteriorate, prompt action must be taken.

Radiological/endoscopic

In favourable cases of abscess formation, (unilocular, well defined), drainage may be performed radiologically. Patients with cholangitis or pyonephrosis due to an obstructed system require urgent decompression. This may be via a radiological or an endoscopic procedure.

Surgical

The aim of surgical intervention is to:

- eliminate the cause of contamination;
- prevent persistent sepsis;

- establish gut integrity, or if not possible, to defunction the bowel (intra-abdominal sepsis);
- ensure adequate drainage and peritoneal toilet.

Control is achieved by resecting or repairing perforated viscera and debriding necrotic tissue. The decision to perform primary repair or defunction the bowel depends on the patient's haemodynamic stability, extent of inflammation, the degree of contamination and the viability of the bowel. A thorough lavage with special attention to the areas where collections commonly form is required together with the appropriate use of drains. The actual surgical procedure will depend on the cause of the sepsis but will adhere to the above principles.

The use of laparoscopy to manage surgical patients with sepsis has been limited due to the concerns regarding haemodynamic compromise and the potentiation of bacteraemia from the pneumoperitoneum using CO_2. It has been effectively employed in the management of acute appendicitis and perforated duodenal ulcer. Bedside diagnostic laparoscopy on Critical Care has been reported as a feasible, safe and accurate method for the assessment of intra-abdominal pathology in critically ill patients.

Sepsis increases the permeability of the gut mucosa, allowing translocation of bacteria and endotoxins, which propagate the septic process. The provision of nutritional support to critically ill patients and maintenance of gut substrates such as glutamine are important supportive measures.

Further reading

Anderson ID, ed. *Care of the Critically Ill Surgical Patient*. Arnold, London, 1999, © The Royal College of Surgeons of England.

Aslam MK & Hunter JD. Necrotising fasciitis. *British Journal of Intensive Care* 2007; **17** (4): 120–125.

Bosscha K, Reijnders K, Hulstaert PF, Algra A & van der Werken C. Prognostic scoring systems to predict outcome in peritonitis and intra-abdominal sepsis. *The British Journal of Surgery* 1997; **84**: 1532–1534.

Marcello PW. Intra-abdominal sepsis. In: O'Donnell JM & Nacul FE, eds. *Surgical Intensive Care Medicine*, Chapter 28. Kluwer Academic Publishers, Massachusetts, USA, 2001: 461–470.

Ordenez CA & Puyana JC. Management of peritonitis in the critically ill patient. *The Surgical Clinics of North America* 2006; **86**: 1323–1349.

CHAPTER 12

Special Cases: The Immunocompromised Patient

Manos Nikolousis

Heart of England NHS Foundation Trust, Birmingham, UK

OVERVIEW

- Sepsis is life threatening in the immunocompromised patient
- Prompt initiation of broad-spectrum antibiotics according to local protocols is crucial
- Appropriate fluid resuscitation and close liaison with Critical Care may improve outcome
- Microbiology advice is essential
- High-risk patients are especially those with an absolute neutrophil count of <500 cells/mm³
- Main source of sepsis is bacterial but fungal and viral pathogens could also lead to severe sepsis and need prompt diagnosis and treatment

---

Introduction

Infection is common in immunocompromised patients and can be rapidly life threatening. Advice should always be sought using local expertise and referral to local guidelines. This demands a multidisciplinary approach depending on the patient and the infection, involving virologists, the Infectious Diseases and Infection Control teams, acute physicians, haematologists, oncologists and the Critical Care team.

Risk factors in immunocompromised patients

Immunocompromised patients have alterations in phagocytic, cellular or humoral immunity that increase both the risk of infection and the ability to combat infection. A patient's immunity may be impaired temporarily or permanently as a result of either an immunodeficiency disease state (congenital or acquired) or induced immunosuppression due to disease management using cytotoxic, immunosuppressive or radiation therapy (for example, to support bone marrow transplantation, solid organ transplantation or malignant diseases) (Tables 12.1–12.3).

The cause of immunodeficiency, and extent and duration of neutropenia, affect the degree of risk of developing infection. There is an inverse relationship between infection risk and absolute neutrophil count. Risk is highest for severe neutropenia (absolute neutrophils <500 cells/ mm³).

Patients who have neutropenia after cytotoxic chemotherapy or immediately after preparative therapy for transplantation nearly always have breaches of physical defense barriers. Mucositis of the oral cavity and gastrointestinal tract permit changes in bacterial flora as well as serving as foci for local infection and entry points for systemic invasion. Such patients are also likely to have alterations in cellular immunity (including drops in CD4 cell counts and function) as well as hypogammaglobulinemia, which make these patients among the most vulnerable to acute infections.

These patients are at high risk of developing overwhelming hospital-acquired infections with opportunistic organisms, and every effort must be made to minimize the risk of transmission of infection. These practices are dealt with in detail in a previous chapter. Barrier nursing becomes of paramount importance.

Table 12.1 Causes of immunodeficiency and categorization of risk.

High risk	Intermediate risk	Low risk
Haematological malignancies	Solid tumours (particularly after cytotoxic chemotherapy)	Long-term corticosteroid use (such as patients with rheumatoid arthritis)
AIDS patients with low CD4+ counts		
Bone marrow transplantation	HIV/AIDS	Diabetic patients
Post-splenectomy patients	Solid organ transplant	Collagen tissue disorders
Genetic disorders such as severe combined immunodeficiency		

AIDS, acquired immunodeficiency disease; HIV, human immuodeficiency virus.

Table 12.2 Definitions of degrees of neutropenia (normal range 1500–2000 cells/mm³).

Mild neutropenia	1000–1500 cells/mm³ (1.0–1.5)
Moderate neutropenia	500–1000 cells/mm³ (0.5–1.0)
Severe neutropenia	<500 cells/mm³ (<0.5)

ABC of Sepsis. Edited by Ron Daniels and Tim Nutbeam. © 2010 by Blackwell Publishing, ISBN: 978-1-4501-8194-5.

Table 12.3 Relation between duration of neutropenia and risk.

Low risk	Neutropenia for <10 d (may have excellent outcome following treatment of infection)
High risk	Neutropenia for >10 d (may have poor outcome following treatment of further infective episodes)

Barrier nursing is the use of infection control practices aimed at controlling the spread of, and eradicating, pathogenic organisms. These practices may require the setting up of mechanical barriers to contain pathogenic organisms within a specified area.

Types of barrier nursing
Source isolation
Designed to prevent the spread of pathogenic microorganisms from an infected patient to other patients, hospital personnel and visitors.

Protective isolation
Protects the patient from the hospital environment. Protective isolation techniques have also been referred to as reverse barrier nursing and reverse isolation and include the use of high-efficiency particulate air (HEPA) filters.

Likely causative organisms

Bacteria
Bacteria represent the most immediate threat to immunocompromised hosts. During the past two decades, there have been changes in the organisms most frequently responsible for infection in immunocompromised neutropenic hosts. Gram-positive organisms, especially coagulase-negative staphylococci, have emerged as the leading cause of acute bacterial infections associated with fever and neutropenia in patients in the United States and Western Europe. The increased prevalence of these organisms may be partly due to the increased use of indwelling intravenous access devices and partly due to injudicious antibiotic prophylaxis and poorly selected therapeutic antibiotic regimes. In addition to coagulase-negative staphylococci, *Staphylococcus aureus* as well as streptococci and enterococci (the latter associated, in some centres, with resistance to vancomycin), are the principal gram-positive isolates, accounting for over half of all microbiologically defined infections in these patients. Enterococci, including vancomycin-resistant enterococci, are a particular problem for patients receiving liver transplants.

In contrast, in developing countries, gram-negative organisms such as *Pseudomonas aeruginosa*, *Escherichia coli* and *Klebsiella* species still predominate, with a pattern similar to that in the United States and Europe in the 1960s and 1970s. Despite their predominance, gram-positive organisms less commonly cause immediately life-threatening infections. The main reason for the prompt evaluation and empirical treatment of immunocompromised patients with bacterial infection is the risk of a more serious untreated infection with gram-negative bacteria.

Patients who are functionally asplenic (for example, from sickle cell disease) or who have had a splenectomy (especially when

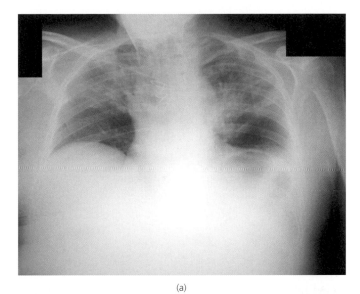

(a)

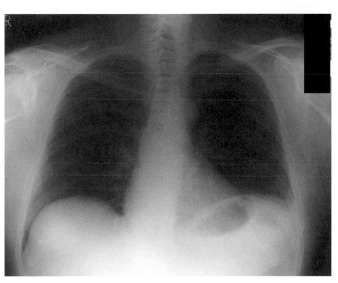

(b)

Figure 12.1 Cytomegalovirus (CMV) pneumonitis (a) pre- and (b) post-treatment – chest radiograph (CXR).

performed because of a malignant disorder, for example, Hodgkin's disease) have increased vulnerability to life-threatening infections with encapsulated bacteria (for example, *Streptococcus pneumoniae*, *Neisseria meningitidis* and *Haemophilus influenzae*). This is particularly true if they have not been immunized. In patients who have undergone splenectomy and in both children and adults infected with the human immunodeficiency virus (HIV), *S. pneumoniae* is the leading bacterial pathogen, and is frequently associated with bacteraemia. Pneumococcal bacteraemia carries a mortality of 20% in this group, with approximately 50% of associated deaths occurring within the first 48 hours of admission. The clinical picture is one of a rapid deterioration to multi-organ failure. Gram-negative organisms, including *P. aeruginosa*, can also cause pneumonia and bacteraemia in patients with acquired immunodeficiency syndrome (AIDS), especially those with low CD4 counts.

Viruses

Patients with neutropenia who have received cytotoxic therapy or bone marrow transplants are also vulnerable to infections with viruses, including herpes viruses and respiratory viruses. Reactivation of dormant viruses can occur in seropositive patients (mainly cytomegalovirus (CMV), herpes simplex virus, herpes zoster virus and Epstein-Barr virus reactivation in patients with haematopoetic bone marrow transplants, solid organ transplants or HIV). Transplant patients who are at the highest risk for CMV reactivation are those who are seropositive with a seronegative donor. Certain viruses can cause acute fever and pneumonia, particularly respiratory syncytial virus, adenovirus, parainfluenza virus and CMV (Figure 12.1). Infections with opportunistic and endemic fungi (see next section) can occur as secondary complications in patients with protracted neutropenia or organ transplant recipients with CMV infection. HIV patients with a high viral load and low CD4 count are susceptible to JC (John Cunningham) virus, which can cause progressive multifocal leucoencephalopathy.

Fungi

Factors including the use of central venous catheters in these patients have also increased the rate of fungal infections by *Candida* or *Aspergillus*. Candida infections have recently been found to be the most frequent infection in patients in Critical Care, and are becoming more diverse. Over the two decades to 1990, non-albicans species represented 10–40% of all candidaemias. In contrast, in 1991–1998, they represented 35–65% of all candidaemias. The most common non-albicans *Candida* species are *Candida parapsilosis* (20–40% of species), *C. tropicalis* (10–30%), *C. krusei* (10–35%) and *C. glabrata* (5–40%). Oral, oesophageal and hepatosplenic candidiasis are frequently seen in immunocompromised patients (Figure 12.2). Invasive aspergillosis is primarily seen in long-term neutropenic patients and, unless neutrophil counts recover, the use of antifungal medication on its own is ineffective.

Finally, in patients with low CD4 (<200 cells/mm^3) counts, or post-bone marrow transplant patients who also have a low CD4 count (<200 cells/mm^3), sepsis can be caused by *Pneumocystis carinii* – a life-threatening opportunistic infection. The taxonomic class of *P. carinii* remains uncertain as it has both fungal and protozoan characteristics. The use of prophylaxis with co-trimoxazole when CD4 count <200 cells/mm^3 significantly reduces the rate of infection by Pneumocystis.

Signs and symptoms

Immunocompromised patients with sepsis usually present in a critical condition. A few of these patients may initially appear clinically well; this can be misleading and sudden deterioration is very common. Even relatively benign causes of immunocompromise such as steroid use can mask symptoms until organ failure is imminent.

Fever, dyspnoea, cough, tachycardia and hypotension with oliguria or anuria are the most common signs of sepsis. In absolute neutropenia, pyrexia may be absent or the patient may be hypothermic. Cutaneous septic emboli may be seen (*S. aureus*), or ecthyma gangrenosum as a cutaneous manifestation of Pseudomonas septicaemia (Figure 12.3). Septic emboli have been described in the brain (especially after infective endocarditis), presenting as confusion, lethargy, ataxia or agitation or with focal neurological signs.

Investigations

First-line investigations for a septic immunocompromised patient include a full set of blood cultures (both peripheral cultures and from a peripheral or central venous catheter if in situ), urine microscopy and culture and a chest X-ray. If there is evidence of pneumonia, sputum cultures should also be requested. If central nervous system sepsis is suspected, a lumbar puncture should be performed using the aseptic technique after excluding the presence of a space-occupying lesion. Samples should be sent for both bacterial and viral analysis (in HIV patients Indian ink stain for *Cryptococcus* is essential). The presence of a wound (for example,

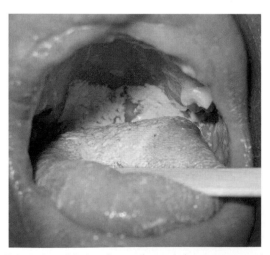

Figure 12.2 Oral candidiasis as frequently seen in immunocompromised patients.

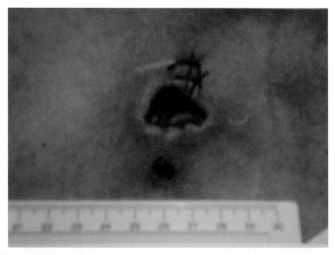

Figure 12.3 Pseudomonas eschar near Hickman line exit in a bone marrow transplant patient.

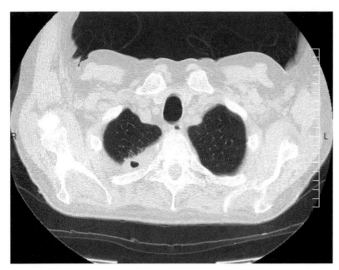

Figure 12.4 A CT scan of the chest showing pulmonary aspergillosis.

leg ulcers in diabetic patients) or inflammation around the central venous catheter should guide the clinician to request a wound or line swab, and to consider the removal of indwelling devices. If the patient develops diarrhoea, stool samples should also be sent for culture.

Blood tests which may be helpful in the investigation and management of such patients include full blood count, biochemistry including renal function and liver function tests, and C-reactive protein.

A clotting screen should also be included in the investigations, as coagulopathy may develop because of intravascular coagulation with consumption of major clotting factors including platelets, excessive fibrinolysis or a combination of both.

When viral infection is strongly suspected (for example, in haematopoetic and solid organ transplants and HIV patients) blood samples should be sent to test for CMV and adenovirus polymerase chain reaction. If flu-like symptoms are present, a nasopharyngeal aspirate should be requested. In transplant patients, CMV reactivation can occur from the second post-transplant week until 6 months post transplant or even later in the presence of graft versus host disease (GvHD).

High-resolution computerized tomography (CT) scan has enabled the early diagnosis of fungal infections, and should be requested if the symptoms do not settle on second-line antibiotics (Figure 12.4). Occasionally, the diagnosis of a fungal infection can prove difficult (if imaging does not lead to a definite conclusion), in which case a bronchioalveolar lavage should be requested. Recent advances have been made in the diagnosis of aspergillosis in the form of the Galactomannan test.

If *Pneumocystis carinii* pneumonia (PCP) is suspected, exercise oxygen saturation should be performed and sputum samples for PCP requested.

Management

The crucial points in the management of sepsis in immunocompromised patients, as in other cases, are the early identification of sepsis,

sampling of diagnostic cultures and the prompt use of antibiotics (Figure 12.5). Attention should also be given to adequate delivery of supplemental oxygen. Different studies have shown that the initiation of antibiotics in the first 30 minutes is crucial in the survival of these patients. Because of the blunted inflammatory response in patients with neutropenia, the signs and symptoms of infection can be minimal, so a heightened index of suspicion for infection is essential.

If the patient is haemodynamically unstable, fluid resuscitation with crystalloid solutions such as Hartmann's, or colloids, should be promptly initiated and the Critical Care Outreach team informed. If the patient does not respond to volume resuscitation, vasoactive drugs may be required. Fluids should be administered cautiously in patients with underlying heart failure. For neutropenic patients, full barrier nursing is extremely important.

First-line antibiotics should include a broad-spectrum antipseudomonal penicillin (such as piperacillin/tazobactam) or, if the patient is allergic, a reasonable alternative would be ceftazidime or a carbapenem (Table 12.4). If chest symptoms are present,

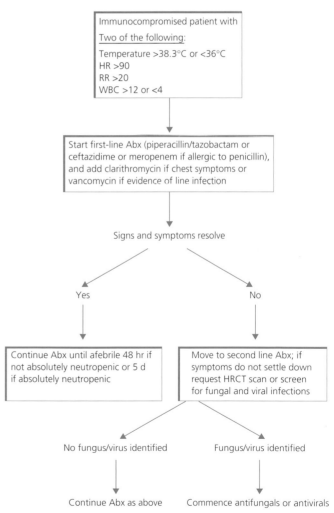

Figure 12.5 An example of an algorithm on the management of sepsis in immunocompromised patients. HR, heart rate; RR, respiratory rate; WBC, white blood cell; Abx, antibiotics; HRCT, high-resolution computerized tomography.

Table 12.4 Microbiological cover spectrum of some major antibiotics in immunocompromised patients.

Piperacillin/ tazobactam	Polymicrobic infections including those with gram-positive and gram-negative aerobic and some anaerobic organisms (intra-abdominal, skin and skin structure, lower respiratory tract)
Carbapenems (imipenem/ meropenem)	Gram-positive and gram-negative aerobic and/or anaerobic organisms. Beta-lactam stable. Better gram-negative cover than piperacillin/tazobactam
Vancomycin	Intravenous: Gram-positive organisms and MRSA PO: Pseudomembranous colitis (relapsed along with metronidazole or alone if metronidazole contraindicated
Metronidazole	Anaerobic cover, pseudomembranous colitis Effective against *Gardnerella*, *Entamoeba histolytica* and *Giardia lamblia*

MRSA, methicillin-resistant *Staphylococcus aureus*.

Table 12.5 Some commonly used antifungal agents.

Standard amphotericin B:
IV dose 1 mg/kg; maximum dose 1.5 mg/kg (very rarely used)
Test dose indicated – 1 mg
Effective against *Candida* and *Aspergillus*
Side effects (often severe): anaphylactic reactions, renal impairment, potassium loss through the gut, arrhythmias

Liposomal amphotericin B:
IV dose 3–5 mg/kg
Effective against *Candida, Aspergillus*; also used in cryptococcal meningitis and visceral leishmaniasis
Side effects: anaphylactic reactions, renal impairment, potassium loss
However, less profound than standard Amphotericin

Echinocandins-caspofungin:
IV dose 70 mg loading, then 50 mg/d if <70 kg or 70 mg/d if >70 kg
Covering all *Candida* species and *Aspergillus*
Side effects: liver impairment, rash

Azoles

Fluconazole
Usually given as prophylaxis
Effective for treatment of oral thrush and oesophageal candidiasis – usually given as 400 mg for 2 d followed by 100 mg for 2 wk
Effective against most *Candida* but not effective for *Aspergillus*
Side effects: hepatic impairment, arrhythmias

Voriconazole
Loading dose 400 mg bd for 3 doses followed by 200 mg bd daily
Oral administration equally effective as IV due to excellent tissue penetration
Effective against both *Candida* and *Aspergillus*
Side effects: hallucinations, liver impairment, visual defects, arrhythmias

Itraconazole
Oral dose 2.5 mg/kg
Effective against Candida but controversial for Aspergillus infection

IV, intravenous.

a macrolide should be considered to cover atypical organisms. Microbiology advice should be sought in order to identify the likely responsible organism and antibiotic sensitivities as well as to determine the duration of treatment. If the fever persists for more than 72 hours on first-line antibiotics, the patient should be switched to second-line antibiotics depending on local guidelines

after checking on cultures and sensitivities. The presence of a central venous catheter should be reported to the microbiology team and consideration given to its removal. Femoral lines are more susceptible to infection than subclavian or jugular central lines. In patients with severe prolonged neutropenia, empirical treatment with antifungals should be initiated and diagnostic imaging targeted to the presumed source requested. If liver function tests are deranged, or liver enzymes elevated, particularly in the absence of positive blood cultures; hepatosplenic candidiasis should be considered and CT of the abdomen is required.

If PCP is diagnosed, high-dose co-trimoxazole 120 mg/kg divided in four doses should be administered and treatment should usually continue for 2 weeks. If PaO$_2$ is <7.0 kPa, a short course of steroids may be beneficial.

As described above, immunocompromised patients are prone to atypical infections with viral and fungal causative agents. A decision to treat empirically using an anti-viral or anti-fungal agent should be based on the individual patient's risk factors and history of previous infections, with perceived benefit balanced against the risks of administering frequently noxious drugs. Tables 12.5 and 12.6 list some of the most commonly used agents in each group. The anti-viral agent Ostelmavir (Tamiflu®, Roche) is currently in use in a number of countries with the aim of symptom reduction in

Table 12.6 Some commonly used antiviral agents.

Aciclovir
Used for the treatment of HSV infection and VZV infection
Usually dose 400 mg five times a day orally for herpes simplex infection or 800 mg five times a day for shingles
IV 10 mg/kg three times daily used for poorly responding patients or herpetic encephalitis

Ganciclovir
Used for treatment of CMV reactivation
IV dose 5 mg/kg twice daily
Side effects: myelosuppression, renal impairment

Foscarnet
Used for treatment of CMV reactivation if severe myelosuppression from ganciclovir or resistant CMV
IV dose 60–90 mg/kg up to 120 mg/kg twice daily depending on creatinine clearance
Side effects: Mainly renal impairment, myelosuppression (less common than ganciclovir), hypokalaemia, hypocalcaemia, hypophosphataemia, renal impairment

Cidofovir
Used for the treatment of CMV reactivation/adenovirus infection
IV dose 5 mg/kg once weekly for the first 2 wk, then every fortnight with concomitant use of probenecid
Side effects: myelosuppression, renal impairment, hepatic toxicity

Ribavirin
Used in aerolized nebulizers 2 g over 2 h three times daily for the treatment of respiratory syncytial virus (RSV)
Side effects: rash, allergic reactions, myelosuppression

Ostelmavir
Used for the treatment of influenza (mainly influenza type B)
Oral dose 75 mg bd

HSV, herpes simplex virus; VZV, varicella zoster virus; IV, intravenous; CMV, cytomegalovirus.

patients with H1N1 influenza ('swine flu') and prophylaxis for their close contacts.

Further reading

Antoniadou A & Giamarellou H. Fever of unknown origin in febrile leukopenia. *Infectious Disease Clinics of North America* 2007; **21** (4): 1055–1090. PMID: 18061089.

Braunwald E, Fauci AS, Kasper DL, Hauser SL, Jameson, JL & Stone RM. *Harrison's Principles of Internal Medicine*, 15th edn, McGraw-Hill, USA, 2001, education ISBN 0071391029.

De Pauw BE. Practical modalities for prevention of fungal infections in cancer patients. *European Journal of Clinical Microbiology and Infectious Diseases* 1997; **16** (1): 32–41. PMID: 9063672.

Glauser M & Pizzo P. *Management of Infections in Immunocompromised Patients*, 1st edn. WB Saunders, 2000, ISBN-10: 0-7020-2506-2.

Pizzo PA. Fever in immunocompromised patients. *New England Journal of Medicine* 2000; **342** (3): 217–218. PMID: 10486422.

Rubin RH & Young LS. *Clinical Approach to Infection in the Compromised Host*, 4th edn. Kluwer Academic/Plenum Publishers, New York, USA 2002, ISBN 0306466937.

CHAPTER 13

The Role of Critical Care

Julian Hull

Good Hope Hospital, Heart of England NHS Foundation Trust, Birmingham, UK

OVERVIEW

- Close, effective communication between the admitting team and Critical Care is vital in severe sepsis

- The Surviving Sepsis Campaign (SSC) has published two internationally recognised 'care bundles' for patients with severe sepsis

- A large component of the 'Resuscitation Bundle', termed early goal-directed therapy (EGDT), strives to optimize tissue oxygen delivery through targeted shock resuscitation

- Support of other organs, including respiratory and renal support, is frequently necessary

- Specific therapeutic interventions, including the use of recombinant activated protein C, may be of benefit

- Consideration should be given in patients not responding to limitation of treatment

---

Severe sepsis (acute organ dysfunction secondary to infection) and septic shock (severe sepsis plus hypotension not reversed with fluid resuscitation) affect millions of individuals around the world each year. Due to its aggressive, multifactorial nature, sepsis is a rapid killer causing death in 30–50% (and often more). This mortality is similar to that of polytrauma, acute myocardial infarction or stroke.

The management of sepsis involves a wide variety of healthcare professionals in its diagnosis and treatment. However, many of those involved outside of the Critical Care environment may not have sufficient training and experience to identify the signs and symptoms of sepsis in order to reach a timely diagnosis, nor to instigate appropriate treatment.

The support and treatment of multiple organ failures resulting from severe sepsis and septic shock is both complex and dynamic, with major changes in therapy often necessary during the first few hours after recognition of the condition.

For these reasons, urgent involvement of the critical care team and subsequent admission to a critical care unit is usually necessary in order to offer the most favourable outcome for patients with severe sepsis.

ABC of Sepsis. Edited by Ron Daniels and Tim Nutbeam. © 2010 by Blackwell Publishing, ISBN: 978-1-4501-8194-5.

General principles

The general care and support of patients with sepsis and a variety of multi-organ failures is underpinned by the well-established **a**irway, **b**reathing, **c**irculation, **d**isability, **e**xposure (ABCDE) approach of assessment and treatment.

Evidence indicates that early goal-directed therapy (EGDT) comprising early sepsis recognition, aggressive resuscitation and therapies, together with appropriate investigation, results in significant reduction in mortality.

The introduction of 'care bundles' can improve outcome by standardizing patient care using multiple evidence-based components bundled together in care plans for specific conditions. Originally pioneered in the United States through the Institute for Healthcare Improvement (IHI) and now supported by the Department of Health, a variety of care bundles are being used in various fields within Critical Care, most notably in sepsis and acute lung injury management (Table 13.1).

Therefore, the point of admission to an intensive care unit (ICU) is a useful time to reassess the patient's whole management up to that point.

With specific regard to patients with sepsis, this means assessing the compliance of treatment with the care bundles recommended by the Surviving Sepsis Campaign (SSC). The SSC care bundles are generally accepted among the international Critical Care community as standards in the treatment of these patients. Care bundles are discussed in further detail in Chapter 16. The SSC has promoted two care bundles: the **Resuscitation Bundle**, to be completed within 6 hours of recognition of treatment, and the **Management Bundle**, to be completed within 24 hours.

Table 13.1 Marked reduction in hospital mortality for patients with severe sepsis when care bundle management is applied.

Compliance with a modified Severe Sepsis Resuscitation Care Bundle	Hospital mortality
Care Bundle Compliant group	23%
Care Bundle Non-compliant group	49% P = 0.01, NNT = 3.9

NNT, Number Needed to Treat. From Gao *et al*. The impact of compliance with 6-hour and 24-hour sepsis bundles on hospital mortality in patients with severe sepsis: a prospective observational study. *Critical Care* 2005; **9**: R764–770.

Continue or establish all elements of the Severe Sepsis Resuscitation Bundle

- Measure serum lactate.
- Obtain blood cultures prior to antibiotic administration.
- Administer broad-spectrum antibiotics.
- In the event of hypotension and/or hypoperfusion start EGDT:
  - Give rapid fluid challenges (initially 20 ml/kg) and achieve central venous pressure (CVP) >8 mmHg.
  - If hypotension remains (mean arterial pressure (MAP) <65 mmHg, systolic blood pressure (SBP) <90 mmHg), administer a vasopressor (noradrenaline infusion or dopamaine) via a central line.
  - If there is evidence of hypoperfusion (ScvO$_2$ <70%), then ensure adequate haemoglobin (check local protocol) and consider inotropic therapy (dobutamine).

Clearly, large components of the resuscitation bundle are applicable outside Critical Care, and should be delivered as soon as possible following recognition of severe sepsis rather than awaiting Critical Care input. Education initiatives are available to aid in completion of these goals, including Survive Sepsis in the United Kingdom.

Continue or establish all elements of the Severe Sepsis Management Bundle

- Inspiratory plateau pressures maintained <30 cmH$_2$O for mechanically ventilated patients.
- Low-dose steroids considered for septic shock refractory to fluids and vasopressors.
- Tight glucose control maintained (suggested <8.3 mmol/l).
- Drotrecogin alfa (activated) suggested for use in patients with high risk of death (not for use in patients with low risk of death).

Specific considerations

Source of infection

Every effort must be made to identify and eradicate the source of infection. This may require urgent ultrasound examination, computerized tomography (CT) or magnetic resonance imaging (MRI) scanning and lead to emergency surgery.

Management

Airway, breathing and ventilation

Many patients develop sepsis following pneumonia. But patients with severe sepsis (with or without pulmonary sepsis) not infrequently develop a spectrum of secondary inflammatory lung injury called acute lung injury (ALI), which in its most severe form, acute respiratory distress syndrome (ARDS), is life threatening. These syndromes manifest as acute respiratory distress, hypoxia, tachypnoea and bilateral pulmonary infiltrates on chest X-ray. Initially this may be managed with high inspired oxygen (FiO$_2$) and continuous positive airway pressure (CPAP) in spontaneously breathing patients (Figure 13.1).

Increasing endothelial and alveolar damage leads to worsening V/Q mismatch, hypoxia and increased work of breathing.

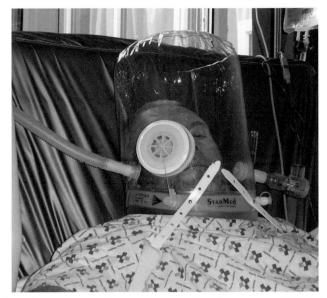

Figure 13.1 Patient receiving continuous positive airway pressure (CPAP) via a hood system (with patient's permission).

Intubation and intermittent positive pressure ventilation (IPPV) are frequently required in response to severe hypoxia and physical exhaustion. Intubation is also required in obtunded patients who are at risk of aspiration.

Once intubated and ventilated, the aim is to provide adequate oxygenation (PaO$_2$ about 10 Kpa) with the lowest FiO$_2$ possible (<0.6, that is, a 60% inspired concentration). An 'open-lung' protective strategy is used to balance improved oxygenation against minimizing ventilator-induced lung injury (VILI). This is achieved by combining alveolar recruitment manoeuvres with high levels of positive end-expiratory pressure (PEEP) (up to 20 cmH$_2$O), to increase the amount of lung which is ventilating and performing gas exchange. This helps to improve oxygenation and also minimize low volume lung injury. 'Safe zone' pressure controlled ventilation with small tidal volumes (approximately 6 ml/kg of ideal body weight) is usually employed to keep peak airway pressures <30 cmH$_2$O (Pmax), thus helping to prevent high-volume lung damage (Figure 13.2). Sometimes this may only be achieved by

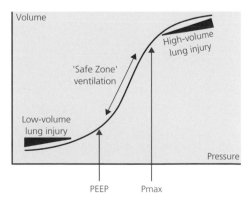

Figure 13.2 Lung compliance curve indicating 'safe' zone for ventilation, areas for lung injury and relevant position of positive end-expiratory pressure (PEEP) and Pmax ventilation pressure limits.

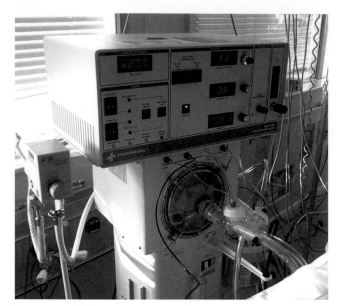

Figure 13.3 High-frequency oscillator ventilator.

allowing a degree of 'permissive' hypercapnia, following a reduction in alveolar ventilation. In other words, it is safe to allow a degree of hypercapnia in order to minimize the risk of VILI occurring.

If hypoxia persists despite ventilation, longer inflation times ('reverse inspiratory time to expiratory time (I:E) ratio') can be used, as well as ventilating the patient in the prone position. The use of high frequency oscillatory ventilation (HFOV) (Figure 13.3), with a respiratory rate around 300/minute, may be beneficial in refractory ARDS patients, with evidence for reduced lung injury.

The respiratory care is usually provided within the framework of a 'Ventilation Care Bundle', which also includes: (Figures 13.4–13.6)

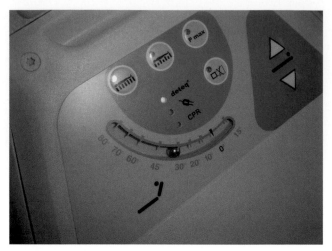

Figure 13.5 Critical Care bed control with inclinometer allowing head up angle measurement.

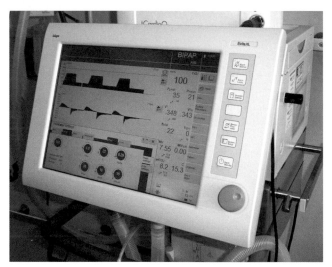

Figure 13.6 Ventilator with pressure-controlled Biphasic Positive Airways Pressure (BiPAP) mode.

- Deep venous thrombosis (DVT) prophylaxis;
- Stress ulcer prophylaxis;
- A 30–40° head-up tilt to reduce gastric regurgitation and ventilator-associated pneumonia (VAP);
- Daily sedation breaks to prevent accumulation of sedative drugs and promote early weaning from ventilation when appropriate.

Vascular access and monitoring

For patients with severe sepsis and septic shock the following are usually considered essential:

- Continuous electrocardiographic (ECG) monitoring;
- Large-bore peripheral venous cannulae for rapid infusion of crystalloids, colloids and blood products as deemed necessary;
- Arterial line for continuous arterial blood pressure (BP) monitoring and blood sampling for initial blood gases, lactate and full blood count (FBC), Urea and electrolytes (U&Es), liver function tests (LFTs), amylase, clotting studies and later repeated tests;

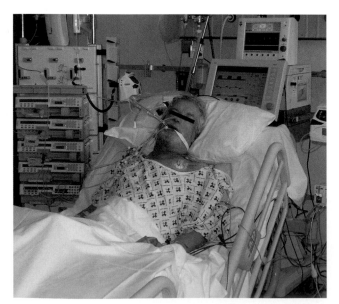

Figure 13.4 Typical patient with severe sepsis undergoing ventilation with 'care bundle' management (with patient's permission).

- Multi-lumen central venous line for CVP measurement, $ScvO_2$ sampling and drug administration – especially vasopressors and inotropes;
- Nasogastric (NG) tube for gastric aspiration and NG feeding;
- Urinary catheter for hourly urine output measurement and sampling for biochemistry and microbiology;
- Continuous SpO_2 monitor;
- Continuous central body temperature.

Aspects related to monitoring are discussed in detail in the next chapter.

Cardiovascular support and early goal-directed therapy (EGDT)

The initial and ongoing fluid resuscitation (EGDT) of patients with severe sepsis and tissue hypoperfusion (hypotension and/or lactate >4 mmol/l) is built around fluid challenges of 20 ml/kg of crystalloid or 10 ml/kg of colloid divided into boluses of 300–500 ml delivered over a maximum of 30 minutes (but as rapidly as possible). These should be repeated based on response until tissue hypoperfusion is relieved or there is evidence of intolerance of fluid resuscitation, that is, a lack of response to further volume loading.

Fluid requirements in septic shock are high. Volumes of up to 60 ml/kg body weight are not unusual – up to 5 litres in an average male. Fluids should be given until:

- circulatory parameters have returned to normal with an improving lactate and adequate CVP;
- there has been no response despite volumes of 60 ml/kg (or colloid equivalent) being given, or
- there is evidence of increasing respiratory distress.

Invasive and non-invasive cardiac output monitoring may be required if the response to resuscitation is poor as detailed above or ventricular dysfunction is present. Techniques used to monitor cardiac output are discussed in the next chapter.

This is the start of the process of EGDT. This should be started as soon as septic shock is recognized and continued within the critical care unit until adequate perfusion, urine output and cardiac output is achieved or the patient ceases to respond effectively.

Suggested parameters for an effective endpoint to resuscitation are given below:

Mean arterial blood pressure >65 mmHg
Improving capillary refill time
Warming of extremities
Urine output >0.5 ml/kg/hour
Improving mental status

A noradrenaline infusion (initially 0.02–0.4 mcg/kg/minute) should be started in the vasodilated, hypotensive patient with sepsis until the MAP is 65–85 mmHg or returned to normal for that patient. An alternative is high-dose dopamine. In patients refractory to noradrenaline, vasopressin (0.01–0.04 iu/minute) may be given, although there is little evidence of improved outcome with this strategy.

If evidence of inadequate cardiac output exists then dobutamine (5–20 mcg/kg/minute) should be given to increase stroke volume and cardiac output (beware of inducing excessive tachycardia). The requirement for this may be identified through a low central venous oxygen saturation ($ScvO_2$, indicating oxygen demand exceeding delivery to tissues, normal >70%) or through direct or indirect cardiac output measurement methods discussed in the next chapter. If the $ScvO_2$ is low, consideration should also be given to the need for transfusion to improve oxygen-carrying capacity.

One EGDT algorithm, employed in the Emergency Department within the first 6 hours, demonstrated absolute mortality reductions of 16% in septic shock. Evidence to support that particular algorithm beyond the first 6 hours is not currently available, though the principles discussed above are sound, generally accepted and recommended by professional bodies worldwide.

The goals in this EGDT algorithm were:

1 CVP >8 mmHg (or >12 mmHg if ventilated)
2 MAP >65 or SBP >90 mmHg
3 $ScvO_2$ >70%

Together with elements of care discussed in Chapter 6, namely blood culture sampling before antibiotics, antibiotic administration within 1 hour and lactate measurement, EGDT completes the SSC's Resuscitation Bundle.

Low-dose steroids

Historically, recommendations regarding the role of steroids in severe sepsis and septic shock have varied considerably and remained controversial. The rationale for steroid use is that some patients with sepsis will have relative adrenal insufficiency. The SSC now recommends that the use of hydrocortisone (up to 300 mg/day) be considered in patients who have refractory shock and remain hypotensive despite both volume loading and vasopressors. If vasopressor requirements cease then steroids can be stopped early. It is not recommended to wait for a stimulation test (usually a short Synacthen test). A recent multi-centre study, the CORTICUS trial, has led some to abandon the use of corticosteroids in sepsis altogether.

Glucose control

In June 2009, in response to the NICE-SUGAR trial, initial guidance from the SSC regarding tight glycaemic control was changed. The international guidance now recommends starting insulin only if the blood glucose exceeds 10 mmol/l (unless the patient is normally diabetic), with no specific recommendation given to a target range. It is important that patients receiving continuous infusion insulin should also receive glucose in some form, either through parenteral or enteral feeding, or via a peripheral glucose infusion. The initial monitoring will need to be more intense requiring 30–60 minute monitoring. After glucose stabilization is achieved, monitoring may be extended to 4 hours. Hypoglycaemia must be avoided and 'sliding scale'-type regimens may have to be adapted to suit individual patients, especially non-diabetic patients.

Activated protein C/drotrecogin alfa (activated)

A key modulator of the thrombin-triggered coagulation response and the endothelium-mediated inflammatory response to sepsis is the activation of protein C. Inactive protein C is activated by a combination of the endothelial surface receptors (thrombin/thrombomodulin receptor and the protein C receptor) to activated protein C, which therefore has immune-modulatory effects in addition to effects on the coagulation cascade.

In patients with severe sepsis, these endothelial receptors are stripped off the surface of the endothelium and can be identified in the circulation leading to decreased capability for activating protein C. Patients with severe sepsis have been shown to have low levels of activated protein C.

Activated protein C when administered in a blinded, randomized fashion to over 1600 patients with severe sepsis and septic shock produced a 6.1% absolute reduction in mortality (Recombinant Human Activated Protein C Worldwide Evaluation in Severe Sepsis (PROWESS) study). Subsequent studies in lower-risk patients failed to demonstrate benefit, and a recent Cochrane review questioned the validity of the original study. Further research is under way to establish the true role and efficacy of this agent.

National Institute for Health and Clinical Excellence (NICE) and the SSC recommend that activated protein C be used in adult patients who have severe sepsis that has resulted in multiple organ failure (that is, two or more major organs have failed) and who are being provided with optimum intensive care support. The use of drotrecogin alfa (activated) should only be initiated and supervised by a specialist consultant with intensive care skills and experience in the care of patients with sepsis.

Nutritional support

Patients with sepsis are often highly catabolic with high protein turnover. Enteral feeding is the preferred route, with nasojejunal feeding a useful option should nasogastric feeding fail. However, gastro-intestinal tract (GIT) dysfunction in patients with sepsis often necessitates the use of parenteral nutrition despite the increased risk of complications.

Acute renal failure and renal replacement therapy (RRT)

Acute renal failure, severe metabolic acidosis and fluid overload are well known complications of severe sepsis with a high associated mortality and can be treated with varying degrees of success with RRT. The development of acute renal failure is an independent predictor of death in patients with sepsis. Usually continuous veno-veno haemo-diafiltration (CVVHDF) is used, although haemodialyis is also effective if tolerated. Severe haemodynamic instability can be precipitated in patients requiring large amounts of inotrope and vasopressor when initiating CVVHFD. The life span of the filter itself can be severely reduced (from days to hours) in patients with severe sepsis, in part due to adsorption of clot degradation products within the filter itself.

Consideration for limitation of support

Where possible, advance care planning, including the communication of likely outcomes and realistic goals of treatment, should be discussed with patients and families.

It may well be in the patient's best interest to make specific decisions regarding the setting of limits to the level of support or the withdrawal of futile supporting modalities.

Infection control in Critical Care

Preventing further infections and sepsis is a paramount concern especially for the vulnerable critically ill patient. Policies regarding healthcare-associated infections need to be adhered to by the whole team. Special attention must be applied to cross infection control measures and hand washing, as well as best practice for invasive procedures to reduce catheter-related blood stream infections (CRBSI).

Further reading

Dellinger RP, Levy MM, Carlet JM *et al.* Surviving Sepsis Campaign: international guidelines for management of severe sepsis and septic shock. *Crit Care Med* 2008; **36**(1): 296–327.

Haraden, C. What is a Care Bundle: Institute for Healthcare Improvement, 2006. www.ihi.org/IHI/Topics/CriticalCare/IntensiveCare/ImprovementStories/WhatIsaBundle.htm [Accessed 9th July 2006].

Leaver S & Evans T. Acute respiratory distress syndrome. *British Medical Journal* 2007; **355**: 389–394.

NCEPOD. An Acute Problem? A report of the National Confidential Enquiry into Patient Outcome and Death, 2005.

NICE. Acutely Ill Patients in Hospital, July 2007.

Pratt R, Pellowe C, Wilson J *et al.* EPIC 2: national evidence-based guidelines for preventing healthcare – associated infections in NHS hospitals in England. *Journal of Hospital Infection* 2007; **655**: S1–S64.

Rivers E, Nguyen B, Havstad S *et al.* Early goal-directed therapy in the treatment of severe sepsis and septic shock. *New England Journal of Medicine* 2001; **345**: 1368–1377.

CHAPTER 14

Monitoring the Septic Patient

David Stanley

Dudley Group of Hospitals, West Midlands, UK

OVERVIEW

- The usefulness of monitoring can only be as good as its interpretation and the subsequent action taken

- Monitors vary in their accuracy, and the parameters they measure vary in their clinical relevance

- Measurement trends are much more useful than absolute values

- There has been a move away from using the invasive pulmonary artery catheter for cardiac output measurement to numerous other less invasive methods requiring less operator skill

- Newer parameters of cardiac output such as stroke volume (SV) and pulse pressure (PP) are being developed. These may be more reliable than some of the traditional methods

---

All patients with sepsis require monitoring, from intermittent vital signs recorded on a general ward through to continuous invasive measurements of cardiac output and oxygenation on the critical care unit. The fundamental importance of monitoring, of whatever sophistication, is to assist in the dynamic assessment of therapy to guide subsequent management.

In the treatment of sepsis, the evidence base for goal-directed therapy means accurate monitoring has acquired extra importance with targeting of certain values. However, monitoring is only as good as its interpretation and subsequent action. It needs emphasizing that monitoring *per se* does not treat the patient with sepsis. It is the clinicians' response to the information produced that determines effectiveness of therapy. Placing a central venous line in a patient with sepsis to measure the central venous pressure (CVP) is in itself of no patient benefit, yet has the potential to do harm. Spending time placing a difficult arterial line, whilst neglecting fluid resuscitation or early antibiotic administration, is unacceptable.

Cardiovascular monitoring

Clinical monitoring

Clinical parameters are often poor predictors of cardiac output and this has driven the development of monitoring devices.

ABC of Sepsis. Edited by Ron Daniels and Tim Nutbeam. © 2010 by Blackwell Publishing, ISBN: 978-1-4501-8194-5.

However, several observations can be useful. A narrow pulse pressure (PP, see below) can indicate hypovolaemia. Metabolic acidosis may be manifest as hyperventilation. Inadequate cerebral perfusion can cause agitation, confusion and reduced consciousness. Reduced renal perfusion causes oliguria or anuria. Pale, cool peripheries with mottled skin and prolonged capillary refill (normal capillary refill is within 2 seconds) indicate inadequate circulation.

High cardiac output is seen in the classical patient with sepsis, producing warm peripheries and bounding pulses. In fact, patients with sepsis in the later stages frequently have low cardiac output manifest as described above.

Electrocardiographic (ECG) monitoring

Continuous electrocardiographic (ECG) monitoring is required as patients with sepsis are prone to arrhythmias, especially atrial fibrillation. If possible, this should include ST-segment monitoring to detect signs of ischaemia.

Non-invasive arterial blood pressure management

The most common devices used for measuring blood pressure use oscillotonometry. These devices are known as DINAMAPs (devices for indirect non-invasive automatic mean arterial pressure). A basic understanding of methods, limitations and inaccuracies is important. A normal blood pressure does not guarantee adequate blood flow and is not a surrogate for it. Direct cardiac output assessment is therefore required when there are doubts about the adequacy of the circulation.

The middle of the cuff bladder is placed over the brachial artery. Alternatively, placing the cuff over the thigh uses the femoral artery for mesurement. The cuff is deflated from a pressure above systolic blood pressure (SBP). Automated time intervals can be set. As soon as cuff pressure drops below SBP, arterial blood flow produces oscillations in the cuff. Sensed by a transducer, a microprocessor records this as the SBP. With further deflation, maximal oscillations occur at the mean arterial blood pressure (MABP). With continued cuff deflation a rapid decrease in oscillations occurs at the diastolic blood pressure (DBP). MABP is the most accurate, DBP the least in determining perfusion pressure (Table 14.1).

Table 14.1 Non-invasive blood pressure monitoring.

Requirements	Limitations	Complications
Fast cuff inflation to prevent venous stasis	Over-reads if cuff too small	Repeated cuff inflation can cause petechial haemorrhage and nerve injury
Slow cuff deflation ~3 mmHg/s allows sufficient measurement time	Over-reads at low pressures, especially when systolic <60 mmHg	
Appropriate cuff size; should cover two-thirds of the upper arm & 40% of circumference width	Under-reads at high pressures	
	Accuracy lessened by arrhythmias, for example, atrial fibrillation	

Invasive arterial blood pressure monitoring

Invasive blood pressure measurement is needed when frequent, real-time and accurate measurements are required (patients with profound hypotension, arrhythmias or requiring inotropes). It also allows beat-to-beat waveform analysis, regular arterial blood gas analysis and permits forms of cardiac output monitoring.

The radial artery (for comfort, in conscious patients use the non-dominant hand) is the most common site of insertion; it is not an end artery and is a relatively easy site familiar to clinicians. In patients with severe sepsis, what is usually a fairly simple procedure can be difficult and time consuming; alternative sites may be needed. Acceptable alternatives are brachial, femoral, ulnar, axillary, dorsalis pedis and posterior tibial arteries. Specific arterial cannulae should be used as they are no wider than 20-gauge with no injection port. Direct cannulation or Seldinger techniques using specially designed cannulae can be used.

Standardized blood pressure is referenced to heart level at the fourth intercostal space, mid-axillary line. Moving away from the heart, SBP increases and DBP falls. So, for example, SBP in the dorsalis pedis is higher than in the aorta, DBP lower. However, MABP only falls slightly. This emphasizes the importance of using MABP as the measured parameter. MABP is also less prone to inaccuracies from damping of the measuring system (Table 14.2 and Figure 14.1).

Central venous pressure (CVP) monitoring

CVP monitoring requires a cannula placed in a large, valveless vein close to the right atrium. The internal jugular and subclavian veins are most commonly used. To prevent erosion through to the pericardium causing tamponade, the tip of the central venous catheter should lie in the distal superior vena cava proximal to the right atrium, the measured pressure equalling that of the right

Table 14.2 Main complications of invasive arterial blood pressure monitoring.

- Haematoma formation
- Distal ischaemia – from air/clot embolus, drug injection
- Infection
- Exsanguination from accidental disconnection
- Damage to neighbouring structures on insertion
- Skin ulceration

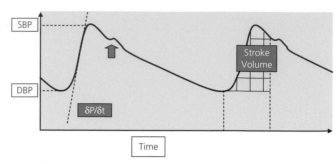

Slope of upslope = δP/δT; directly related to myocardial contractility;
Steep downslope = low SVR
The dicrotic notch (arrowed) is produced by aortic valve closure.
A low relative position on the downslope suggests hypovolaemia.
Wide pulse pressure = low SVR (common in sepsis), aortic regurgitation
Narrow pulse pressure = hypovolaemia, aortic stenosis, damping of the trace (clot, wrist flexed etc.)
Stroke volume is inferred by the area under the curve during systole (hatched area). This is the basis for SV estimation used in pulse contour analysis devices.

Figure 14.1 Arterial waveform and information.

Table 14.3 Recognized complications of central venous pressure (CVP) monitoring.

Early	Late
Arterial puncture – haematoma, arterial insufficiency	Catheter-related bloodstream infection
Pneumothorax, surgical emphysema	Thrombosis
Arrhythmias	Disconnection
Air embolism	Tamponade
Nerve injury – brachial plexus, phrenic	SVC erosion
Tracheal injury	
Thoracic duct injury	

SVC, superior vena cava.

atrium. On a chest X-ray correct placement is confirmed when the line tip is seen lying adjacent to the carina (Table 14.3).

CVP is measured at the end of expiration with the patient lying flat, and referenced against the level of the right atrium, taken as the mid-axillary line. Normal values in spontaneously breathing patients are 4–8 mmHg.

End-diastolic right atrial pressure equals right ventricular end-diastolic pressure (except in tricuspid valve disease). From this, right ventricular end-diastolic volume is inferred and used as a measure of right ventricular pre-load, that is, a measurement of a patient's volume status.

The Surviving Sepsis Campaign guidelines target specific CVP values as a guide to adequate fluid resuscitation. However, in common with much in clinical practice there are numerous situations when this attractively simple assumption is incorrect and CVP is unreliable (Tables 14.4 and 14.5). There is increasing recognition that CVP is actually a poor indicator of a patient's volume loading and status. For example, the application of continuous positive airway pressure (CPAP) or positive end-expiratory pressure (PEEP) reduces right ventricular pre-load causing cardiac output to fall, yet CVP rises. This rise could be taken as an indication that the patient has been adequately fluid resuscitated when this may not be the

Table 14.4 Conditions in which central venous pressure (CVP) measurement is unreliable as a surrogate marker of left ventrivular (LV) pre-load.

- Right ventricular failure
- Tricuspid valve abnormalities
- Pulmonary hypertension
- Pulmonary embolism
- LV hypertrophy
- Myocardial infarction
- Positive end-expiratory pressure (PEEP)

Table 14.5 Rough-guide to central venous pressure (CVP) interpretation of fluid status.

CVP	Patient's volaemic status
Low	↓
Normal	→, ↓
High	↑, →, ↓

↓ = underfilled; → = adequately filled; ↑ = overfilled.

case. As with all monitoring, therefore, values should be interpreted in the context of the clinical findings.

Despite these reservations, measurement of CVP remains the most readily obtainable target for fluid resuscitation. Emphasis must be on use for dynamic measurements, with attention to the magnitude and duration of the change in response to a fluid challenge.

Cardiac output monitoring

Pulmonary artery flotation catheter (PAFC, Swann-Ganz)

Pulmonary artery flotation catheters (PAFCs) are long lines containing three lumens with a thermistor and 2-ml balloon situated at the tip. Inserted via a central vein, they are then 'floated' into a pulmonary artery using the inflated balloon. Using a technique known as thermodilution, a known volume of cold saline is injected via a proximal port located in the right atrium. As this fluid passes the tip of the PAFC in the pulmonary artery, the resulting change in temperature is measured by a thermistor. Using an algorithm the cardiac output can be calculated from the speed with which the cold solution is dissipated.

PAFCs are also used to measure pulmonary artery and pulmonary artery occlusion pressures (PAOPs or 'wedge'). Occlusion pressure is taken as a surrogate marker for left atrial pressure, which at the end of diastole equals left ventricular end-diastolic pressure. In normal situations, this reflects left ventricular end-diastolic volume and therefore left-ventricular pre-load. Clinically, like CVP there are many limitations to these assumptions. Again, despite these reservations these pressure measurements are useful to guide therapy. It allows other indices such as systemic and pulmonary vascular resistance to be calculated.

The PAFC has been the gold-standard monitor of cardiac output against which subsequent devices are measured. However, use is declining with the development of alternative devices, reduced familiarity and skills in its use and controversy over its safety profile.

Oesophageal Doppler

The oesophageal Doppler (OD) consists of a probe inserted via the mouth or nose into the distal oesophagus where the tip lies immediately parallel to the thoracic aorta. It uses the Doppler effect to measure aortic blood flow. The display produced is used to derive stroke volume (SV), and various parameters are calculated.

It is often used in patient optimization when used as part of a fluid management protocol. Typically this consists of administering rapid fluid challenges, for example, giving 250 ml of fluid over 5 minutes and then re-assessing, specifically in terms of SV and flow time corrected (FTc) (Table 14.6 and Figure 14.2).

Arterial waveform analysis

Several devices use a method known as arterial waveform or pulse contour analysis to measure cardiac output. Area under the arterial waveform is analysed and from this the area of systolic ejection produced, permitting calculation of SV. It is less reliable when arrhythmias are present as identification of closure of the aortic valve is required (indicated by the dicrotic notch). SV variation is one of the parameters produced and displayed.

Pulse pressure and stroke volume variation

PP is the difference between SBP and DBP (PP = SBP − DBP). During positive-pressure ventilation it changes with each respiratory cycle. This variation increases proportionally to the degree of

Table 14.6 Oesophageal Doppler terminology.

- SV (stroke volume) = volume of blood ejected during systole (ml)
- FTc (flow time corrected) — time of ejection; opening to closing of aortic valve, corrected for heart rate. Flow time naturally reduces with increasing heart rate and correcting this time allows compensation for this
- PV (peak velocity) = peak velocity of blood flow during systole. Measured in cm/s. Corresponds with the maximal height of the wave on the display. Declines with patient age. An indicator of left ventricular contractility
- MA (mean acceleration) = average acceleration of blood flow from onset of systole to the peak velocity. Corresponds with the steepness of the upslope of the wave. An indicator of left ventricular contractility
- CI (cardiac index) = cardiac output adjusted for body surface area.
- SVR (systemic vascular resistance) = the resistance against which the left heart pumps; left ventricular afterload.

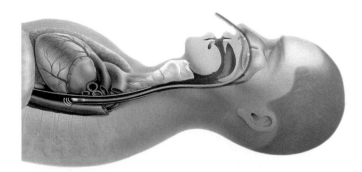

Figure 14.2 Oesophageal Doppler in-situ. (Reproduced with permission from Deltex Medical.)

Table 14.7 Methods of measuring cardiac output in routine use.

	Central venous cannulation required	Arterial cannulation required	Invasive	Continuous measurement possible	Operator skill/training required	Validated against PAFC
Pulmonary artery catheter	Yes	No	Yes	Yes	Medium/high	
Oesophageal Doppler	No	No	Semi	Yes	Low	Yes
Echocardiography	No	No	Semi, if TOE	No	High	Yes
PiCCO	Yes	Specific arterial line placed in brachial or femoral	Yes	Yes	Low/medium	Yes
LiDCO	No	Standard radial arterial line	Yes	Yes	Low	Yes
FloTrac-Vigileo	No	Standard radial arterial line	Yes	Yes	Low	No – imprecise but follows trends accurately

hypovolaemia. Therefore, measuring this change, known as pulse pressure variation (PPV), is useful in monitoring the volaemic states of patients with sepsis. Shown to be an excellent predictor of fluid responsiveness in patients with sepsis, PPV is defined as the maximal and minimum PP divided by the mean of these two values. A value >13% suggests hypovolaemia requiring fluid. Studies show PPV to be far superior to CVP and PAOP in predicting fluid responsiveness.

Stroke volume variation (SVV) is similar in principle to PPV, measuring the respiratory variation of SV. It is defined as the difference between the maximal and minimum SV during one mechanical breath divided by the mean SV.

There are several monitors displaying PPV or SVV (for example, PiCCO, LiDCO, Vigileo). Unfortunately, the major limitation to use of these parameters is the need for patients to be fully ventilated; any spontaneous respiratory effort invalidates PPV and SVV as reliable parameters. Likewise, these parameters are inaccurate in certain conditions, for example, left ventricular failure, arrhythmias. Individual devices are of different precision (Figure 14.3).

Echocardiography

Transthoracic echocardiography (TTE) and transoesophageal echocardiography (TOE) are increasingly used to assess haemo-dynamics in critically ill patients with sepsis. In addition, other useful information can be gained which often influences ongoing

management, for example, evidence of valvular heart problems and pulmonary embolism.

The range devices used in the measurement of cardiac output is summarised in Table 14.7.

Other devices

Pulse oximetry

Pulse oximetry is invaluable in managing the patient with sepsis. Placed on the finger, toe, ear or nose, it indicates the degree of oxygenation of arteriolar blood. However, it gives no information on actual oxygen delivery to tissues because it does not attempt to measure blood flow.

The oximeter contains two light-emitting diodes and a photode-tector. As oxyhaemoglobin and de-oxyhaemoglobin absorb light of different wavelengths, the oximeter is able to calculate the percentage of oxygenated (saturated) haemoglobin. A trace of blood flow in the monitored part is also displayed (Table 14.8).

Blood tests

Central/mixed venous oxygenation

The oxygen saturation of blood in a central vein is known as central venous saturation ($ScvO_2$). Superior vena cava samples from a central line placed in the internal jugular, subclavian or axillary vein can be taken. Inferior vena cava samples from a femoral line should not be used for $ScvO_2$ measurements as suitable target levels are much less predictable and have not been defined.

Taken from a pulmonary artery via a PAFC, the oxygen saturation is known as the mixed venous saturation (SvO_2). Studies of patients

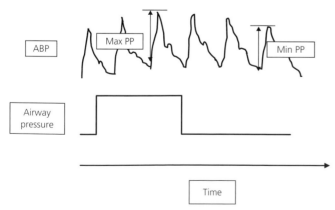

Figure 14.3 Systolic and pulse pressure variation.

Table 14.8 Limitations of pulse oximetry in sepsis.

- Low cardiac output states – check to ensure waveform displayed is consistent with a normal pulsatile waveform. Otherwise, may give falsely low reading
- Readings are averaged over 10–20 s. Any desaturation will have a delay of at least 10–20 s before appearing. Central desaturation takes approximately 60 s to be detected peripherally using a finger probe
- Provides no information on a patient's carbon dioxide levels and therefore is not a monitor of the adequacy of ventilation

with shock indicate that SvO_2 is 5–7% lower than central venous oxygen saturation ($ScvO_2$). When using goal-directed therapy in the patient with sepsis, the target for SvO_2 is therefore >65% as opposed to >70% for $ScvO_2$. Devices are available that allow for continuous measurement of SvO_2.

If the $ScvO_2$ or SvO_2 is low, this implies either that the tissues are extracting more oxygen per unit volume of blood than is normal or that the oxygen content of arterial blood is abnormally low. If the patient is adequately oxygenated i.e. measured oxygen saturations are normal, then oxygen delivery to the tissues is deemed to be inadequate, either due to poor carriage (anaemia) or to low cardiac output.

Lactate

Lactate is produced in excess under anaerobic conditions where it acts as a marker of inadequate tissue perfusion. In sepsis, hyper-lactaemia is mainly due to muscle Na/K adenosine triphosphatase (ATPase) activity. Monitoring its level should be undertaken as soon as sepsis is recognized and trends can guide the adequacy of treatment, especially in the initial resuscitation stage. Normal range is 0–2 mmol/l, levels greater than 4 are independent predictors of poor outcome (mortality >40%). Raised lactate is often seen out of proportion to the clinical condition if adrenaline (epinephrine) is being used as an inotrope.

Inflammatory markers

The white cell count (WCC) is often abnormal in sepsis (WCC <4 or >12 is a criterion of systemic inflammatory response syndrome (SIRS)) and can give clues to origin (neutrophilia suggests bacterial infection). C-reactive protein is an acute phase protein which rises with inflammation of any cause; it is very non-specific. The hormone pro-calcitonin rises in sepsis but only once shock is established-there is some evidence that PCT is more specific to sepsis than CRP. Levels can be used to determine duration of therapy. All these tests assist in the dynamic monitoring of the sepsis treatment response.

Coagulation

With increasing severity of sepsis, abnormalities of clotting are seen ranging from mild elevation in international normalized ratio (INR) and activated partial thromboplastin time (aPTT) through to florid disseminated intravascular coagulopathy (DIC) (markedly elevated INR, APTT and D-dimer, decreased platelets and fibrinogen, presence of fibrin-degradation products).

Further reading

Allsager C & Swanevelder J. Measuring cardiac output. *Continuing Education in Anaesthesia, Critical Care and Pain* 2003; **3**: 15–19.

Al-Shaikh B & Stacey S. *Essentials of Anaesthetic Equipment*, 3rd edn. Churchill Livingstone, London, 2007.

Bersten A, Soni N & Oh T. *Oh's Intensive Care Manual*. Elsevier, London, 2003.

Michard F. Changes in arterial pressure during mechanical ventilation. *Anaesthesiology* 2005; **103**: 419–428.

Wigfull J & Cohen A. Critical assessment of haemodynamic data. *Continuing Education in Anaesthesia, Critical Care and Pain* 2005; **5**: 84–88.

Yentis S, Hirsch N & Mills G. *Anaesthesia and Intensive Care A-Z*, 3rd edn. Butterworth-Heinemann, London, 2004.

CHAPTER 15

Novel Therapies in Sepsis

Gavin D. Perkins[1] *and David R. Thickett*[2]

[1]University of Warwick Medical School, Heart of England NHS Trust, Birmingham, UK
[2]University of Birmingham, University Hospitals Birmingham, Birmingham, UK

OVERVIEW

- A large number of novel therapies for the treatment of sepsis are currently under evaluation

- Novel therapeutic targets include modulation of host pathogen interaction; inflammatory cascade, coagulation/fibrinolysis pathway, microcirculation and apoptosis

- Developments in the field of pharmacogenomics (the influence of genetic variation on drug responses) are likely to play a growing role in selecting the optimal treatment for an individual with severe sepsis

- A number of drugs are undergoing evaluation in clinical trials at present. These include intravenous immunoglobulins, β_2-agonists, statins and high mobility group box protein (HMGB-1) inhibitors.

Box 15.1 **Promising therapeutic targets and agents in sepsis**

Tumour necrosis factor (TNF) neutralizers
    for example, polyclonal anti-TNF antibody
Interleukin (IL)-27 neutralization
    soluble IL-27 receptor fusion protein
Vascular endothelial growth factor (VEGF)
    soluble VEGF receptor 1
Toll-receptor antagonist/signalling
    E5564, TAK-242
Modulation of apoptosis
    Inhibition of Fas-mediated apoptosis by small interfering RNA
Blockade of high mobility group box protein 1 (HMGB-1)
    ethyl pyruvate, anti-HMGB-1 antibody
3-hydroxy-3-methylglutaryl-coenzyme A (HMG-CoA) reductase inhibitors
    statins
Oestrogen receptor beta agonist
    WAY-202196
Oxidants
    N-acetlycysteine
Coagulation
    tissue factor antagonists, anti-thrombin III

Background

Sepsis is a complex, multifactorial syndrome that can develop into conditions of varying severity, ranging from severe sepsis with one-organ failure to multi-organ failure. Significant advances have been made in defining new approaches to the treatment of sepsis in the past decade. These include the use of tight glycaemic control, early goal directed therapy (EGDT) and activated protein C to mention but a few. The development of international guidelines for sepsis in the form of the Surviving Sepsis Campaign and use of sepsis care bundles are contributing to improved outcomes for patients with sepsis. In parallel with these developments, improvements in our understanding of the pathophysiological processes involved in sepsis are helping to open up new avenues for exploring therapeutic interventions. Potential novel targets for drug therapy are outlined in Box 15.1.

Despite these developments, the last 30 years of research into sepsis have delivered only a limited number of new therapies into the clinical arena. A systematic review of 72 large-scale multi-centre studies undertaken in the last decade revealed that only 10 of these trials demonstrated a significant reduction in mortality. Currently there are 491 trials involving sepsis registered with

www.clinicaltrials.gov: 52 phase III trials and 53 phase II trials are currently recruiting as of June 2009. There are several challenges faced by sepsis trials. The first is the difficulty in defining the precise onset of sepsis. The lack of specificity of the current definition and sometimes transient nature of physiological signs contribute to the substantial variability seen between clinicians when determining the onset of sepsis. Further challenges are the huge heterogeneity of the population of patients labelled as having sepsis syndrome. Patients with a diverse range of infecting organisms with varying virulence, different anatomical sites of infection and wide range of host inflammatory and immunologic responses tend to be grouped together in many trials. Future trials may benefit from targeting more homogeneous populations of patients with specific infections (for example, pneumonia) or from targeting patients with specific deficits in the response to infection (for example, protein C levels).

The characteristics of an ideal therapeutic agent for sepsis are outlined in Box 15.2. This chapter will discuss some of the emerging concepts and therapies in the treatment of sepsis.

ABC of Sepsis. Edited by Ron Daniels and Tim Nutbeam. © 2010 by Blackwell Publishing, ISBN: 978-1-4501-8194-5.

Box 15.2 **The characteristics of an ideal therapeutic agent**

Simple dosing regime

Multiple routes of administration – intravenous (IV) and oral/via nasogastric tube

Pleotropic effects upon the inflammatory or coagulant cascade

Minimal side effect profile

Lack of interactions with drugs commonly co-prescribed in sepsis, for example, antibiotics

Effective for a broad range of causative organisms

Inexpensive

Genetic influences

Observational studies in the late 1980s demonstrated that genetic factors play a major part in determining the outcome from sepsis. Advances in genotyping techniques have led to the discovery of single nucleotide polymorphisms (DNA sequence variations that occur when a single nucleotide (A, T, C or G) in the genome sequence is altered) in many of the genes responsible for the host response to infection. These include alterations in tumour necrosis factor-α (TNF-α) and interleukin (IL)-1 receptors, coagulation factors and toll-like receptors. Polymorphisms in cytokine genes may determine the concentrations of inflammatory and anti-inflammatory cytokines an individual produces, and may influence whether someone has hyper-inflammatory or hypo-inflammatory responses to infection. For example, the risk of death among patients with sepsis has been linked to genetic polymorphisms for TNF-α and TNF-β. This genetic variation may also influence the efficacy or toxicity of specific drug interventions in the patient with sepsis.

Collaborative multi-centre observational studies examining the epidemiology of gene polymorphisms (for example, genetics of sepsis and septic shock (GenOSept)) and their influence upon sepsis-related morbidity and mortality are currently in progress. The identification of specific genetic polymorphisms that can predict an individual's response to sepsis and the associated risk of death are likely to lead to individualized and targeted treatment. Future therapeutic trials designed to target specific genotypes and associated cellular responses may help to maximize the clinical response to treatment whilst at the same time maintaining patient safety (pharmacogenomics).

Specific treatments

Polyclonal immunoglobulins

Trials evaluating the role of polyclonal intravenous immunoglobulins (IVIG) date back to the early 1980s. IVIGs possess a number of immunomodulatory properties that may be helpful in improving outcomes in patients with sepsis. The mechanisms of action of IVIG in sepsis involve several pathways in the inflammatory cascade. Experimental studies have shown that IVIGs can enhance bacterial opsonisation ('labelling' of bacteria with plasma proteins to facilitate phagocytosis), phagocytosis and bacterial lysis by the complement system. IVIGs also scavenge activated complement factors, which can reduce complement-mediated tissue damage, modulate cytokine and cytokine antagonist production and neutralize endotoxins (lipopolysaccharide of gram-negative bacteria) and toxins (superantigens of gram-positive bacteria).

The use of varying doses and types of IVIG has been the subject of over 25 clinical trials. However, many of the early trials were of poor quality and lacked sufficient power to detect meaningful differences between groups. The trials to date have principally investigated two different types of IVIG – those containing purely immunoglobulin G (IgG) ('standard' IVIG) or IgM-enriched (Figure 15.1). The IgM-enriched IVIG is considered as more physiological as it reflects

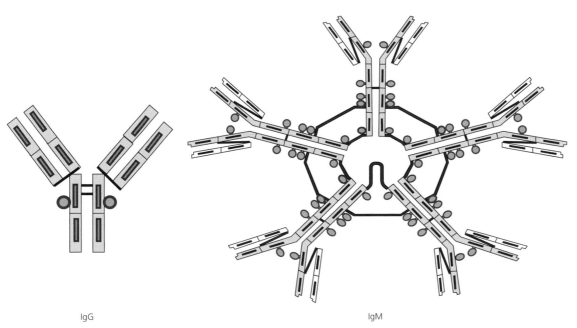

IgG   IgM

Figure 15.1 Immunoglobulin (Ig)M-enriched immunoglobulin is more effective than immunoglobulin solutions containing IgG alone. Pentaglobin is currently the only commercially available IgM-enriched immunoglobulin. It consists of a mixture of IgG: 38 mg/ml (76%), IgM: 6 mg/ml (12%), IgA: 6 mg/ml (12%).

the primary response to infection in humans. The pentameric structure of IgM contributes to a superior efficacy in toxin neutralization and bacterial agglutination compared with IgG antibodies.

At least eight systematic reviews of IVIG for sepsis and septic shock have been published, the earliest in 2002 and the latest in 2007. There are important differences in the conclusions about the effectiveness of IVIG and their recommendations about its use in clinical practice. At one extreme, a review concludes that 'these results should be sufficient reason to use IVIG for adjunctive therapy of severe sepsis or septic shock,' whereas other reviews more cautiously conclude that large, high-quality trials are needed. There remains disagreement over whether benefit from IVIG has been clearly established for any group of patients or for any specific type of IVIG. Few large trials have been conducted (only one of more than 500 patients in adults) and all of the reviews are therefore based mainly or entirely on small trials. It is well known that small trials may be more susceptible to biases, including publication bias, and there is therefore a possibility that meta-analyses will overestimate the treatment effect of IVIG. There are several well-documented examples where meta-analyses of small trials apparently showed convincing benefit, but this was not confirmed by subsequent large randomized trials (for example, aspirin for pre-eclampsia). The situation is further compounded by an international shortage of IVIG. Increasing the use of IVIG for patients with sepsis would further limit availability for other indications. In light of these uncertainties, the UK Health Technology Assessment has recently called for a detailed review of evidence and assessment of the need for a definitive trial.

Do statins have a role in preventing or treating sepsis?

Statins are a class of lipid-lowering drugs. All statin drugs inhibit the enzyme 3-hydroxy-3-methylglutaryl-coenzyme A (HMG-CoA) reductase. HMG-CoA reductase catalyses the conversion of hydroxymethylglutaryl-CoA to mevalonate, an early step in cholesterol synthesis. Inhibition of this enzyme therefore contributes to lowering cholesterol levels. Over the last decade, HMG-CoA reductase inhibitors have emerged as potentially powerful inhibitors of the inflammatory process (Figure 15.2).

The mechanism by which statins modulate the immune response is complex, but is often regarded as lipid independent as it is not related to a lowering of low-density lipoprotein (LDL)-cholesterol. Nevertheless, these effects primarily involve the inhibition of isoprenoid lipid production and subsequent protein prenylation and activation of signalling proteins such as the small guanosine triphosphatase (GTPases).

Support for the anti-inflammatory effects of statins come from in vitro cell culture experiments and animal models of sepsis. Clinical data also supports a beneficial role in sepsis but this data mainly relates to database or retrospective cohort studies. Several single-centre studies are actively recruiting to randomized phase II and III trials to assess the safety tolerability. Currently, however, none of these trials has mortality as an outcome – something that would certainly require a large multi-centre study.

In summary, therefore, there is considerable circumstantial evidence from retrospective database enquiries and observational

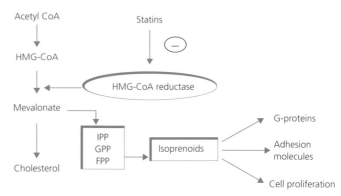

Figure 15.2 Mechanisms of action of statins. HMG-COA, 3-hydroxy-3-methylglutaryl-coenzyme A. IPP, isopentenyl pyrophosphate; GPP. geranyl pyrophosphate; FPP, farnesyl pyrophosphate. Reproduced with permission from Thickett DR, *British Journal of Anaesthesia* 2008; **100** (3): 288–298.

studies that statins may be helpful in sepsis. However, these studies do not explain why the incidence of sepsis is increasing despite rising use of statins in the population and all of these studies have methodological flaws that mean they are poor surrogates for randomised controlled trials.

β_2-Agonists

Experimental studies have shown that β_2-agonists reduce the production of inflammatory cytokines (for example, TNF, IL-8) and free radicals (nitric oxide, superoxide) leading to a reduction in circulating and organ-specific cytokine production. In animal and human volunteer models of sepsis, pre- or early treatment (prior to or shortly after insult) with β_2-agonists has been shown to reduce inflammatory cytokine production, improve coagulation and fibrinolysis profiles and endothelial function, leading to a reduction in organ dysfunction (renal, hepatic, brain). Acute lung injury (ALI) and the acute respiratory distress syndrome (ARDS) are common consequences of severe sepsis. β_2-Agonists may have a special role in the treatment of patients with ALI/ARDS as they have been shown to accelerate intrinsic alveolar fluid clearance mechanisms, potentially leading to early resolution of pulmonary oedema (Figure 15.3). They have also been shown to improve muco-ciliary clearance, increase surfactant processing and release, protect the respiratory epithelium against bacterial-mediated damage and may have a role in promoting repair of the injured lung (Figure 15.4).

Clinical studies using β_2-agonists in humans with sepsis are limited. A single-centre randomized controlled trial (Beta agonists in lung injury (BALTI-1) study) demonstrated that treating patients with ARDS, a common complication of systemic sepsis, with intravenous salbutamol reduced extra-vascular lung water and improved pulmonary mechanics(Figure 15.5). The potential impact of this therapy on patient survival is now being examined in a Medical Research Council (MRC)-funded multi-centre clinical trial of intravenous beta agonists in the United Kingdom (BALTI-2).

High mobility group box protein 1 (HMGB-1)

High mobility group box protein 1 (HMGB-1) is an essential nuclear DNA-binding protein that is a potent pro-inflammatory

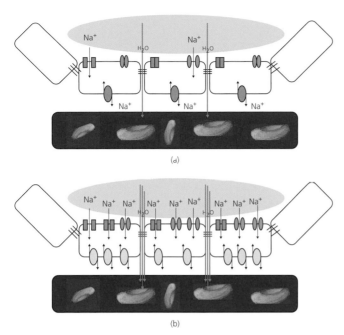

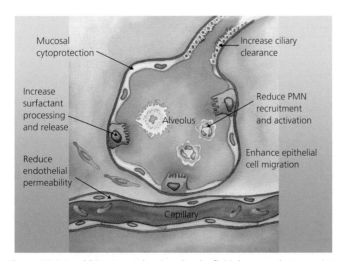

Figure 15.3 Acute lung injury and acute respiratory distress syndrome (ARDS) are characterized by the development of non-cardiogenic pulmonary oedema. This figure is a schematic of the alveolar-capillary unit. (a) Alveolar fluid clearance is driven by the active transport of sodium across the alveolar epithelium. (b) Beta agonists accelerate alveolar fluid clearance by increasing basolateral Na/K adenosine triphosphatase (ATPase) expression and activity, increasing apical Na channel expression and apical Na channel activity leading to a net increase in vectorial Na transport and fluid clearance.

mediator. Unlike several of the early response cytokines such as IL-1 and TNF-α, its secretion appears late in the process of the development of sepsis. Animal models have shown that infusions of HMGB-1 mimic sepsis, and blockade of HMGB-1 reduces organ failure and death. Human studies also demonstrate

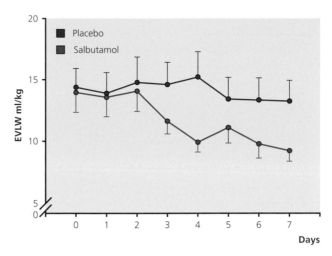

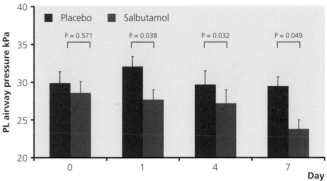

Figure 15.5 Beta agonists reduced extra-vascular lung water (EVLW) and improved lung mechanics in a single-centre trial of intravenous beta agonists in the acute respiratory distress syndrome. With permission from Perkins GD et al. *American Journal of Respiratory and Critical Care Medicine* 2006.

elevated levels of HMGB-1 in patients destined to die as opposed to survivors, making targeting this pathway highly attractive for sepsis therapy.

Several potential strategies for blocking HMGB-1 are under development (Figure 15.6). Ethyl pyruvate, derived from the endogenous metabolite pyruvic acid, has already been investigated in phase 1 studies in man, and in animal studies significantly reduces HMGB-1 levels in sepsis with improved outcome even when given 24 hours after its onset – an important quality for a potential drug treatment for sepsis.

Conclusion

Current therapy for sepsis remains unsatisfactory despite considerable efforts at new drug development. It is important to realize when considering drugs that target the inflammatory cascade that cytokines interact as networks with considerable redundancy of function i.e., blockade of many of the pathways will have little or no effect. Key challenges facing biomedical scientists in developing novel therapies for sepsis include the identification of the central components of these networks, and the determination of which points are amenable to therapeutic targeting to generate drugs that are ideally both effective and specific.

Figure 15.4 In addition to accelerating alveolar fluid clearance, beta agonists may have a number of additional beneficial effects on the alveolar-capillary unit in acute respiratory distress syndrome (ARDS). PMN, polymorph nuclear cells. Source acknowledgement: Perkins GD, McAuley DF, Richter A, Thickett DR & Gao F. Bench-to-bedside review: β2-Agonists and the acute respiratory distress syndrome. *Critical Care* 2004; **8** (1): 25–32. Figure 1.

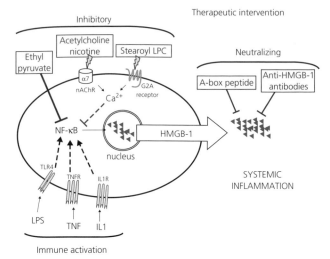

Figure 15.6 Therapeutic targets for high mobility group box protein (HMGB-1) inhibition. With permission from Mantell LL, Parrish WR & Ulloa L. *Shock* 2006.

Progress in the sepsis field could also be enhanced if positive results from preclinical trials using an animal model were predictive of results in humans – sadly, too often this is not the case.

Equally, the search for a reliable biomarker that could be used to target therapy in humans continues. However, even without improvements in preclinical modelling or in the clinical diagnosis of severe sepsis, it seems highly probable that the therapeutic options for treating this life-threatening condition will soon improve.

Further reading

Angus DC & Mira JP. Improving clinical trials in the critically ill: report of a roundtable conference in Brussels, Belgium, March 2008. *Critical Care Medicine* 2009; **37** (1)(suppl): S1–S178.

Cariou A, Chiche JD, Charpentier J, Dhainaut JF & Mira JP. The era of genomics: impact on sepsis clinical trial design. *Critical Care Medicine* 2002; **30** (Suppl 5): S341–S348.

Gao F, Linhartova L, Johnston AM & Thickett DR. Statins and sepsis. *British Journal of Anaesthesia* 2008; **100** (3): 288–298.

Mantell LL, Parrish WR & Ulloa L. Hmgb-1 as a therapeutic target for infectious and inflammatory disorders. *Shock* 2006; **25** (1): 4–11.

Perkins GD, McAuley DF, Richter A, Thickett DR & Gao F. Bench-to-bedside review: beta2-Agonists and the acute respiratory distress syndrome. *Critical Care* 2004; **8** (1): 25–32.

Russell JA. Management of sepsis. *New England Journal of Medicine* 2006; **355** (16): 1699–1713.

CHAPTER 16

Approaches to Achieve Change

Julian F. Bion[1] and Gordon D. Rubenfield[2]

[1]University of Birmingham, University Hospitals Birmingham, Birmingham, UK
[2]Sunnybrook Health Sciences Centre, University of Toronto, Canada

---

OVERVIEW

- Health systems quality improvement (QI) means improving reliability of delivery of best practice care

- Improving reliability of delivery requires changes in clinical behaviour

- Changing behaviour requires rigorous methodologies, research investment and time

- Engagement of front-line staff is central to the success of all QI initiatives

- QI is an integral part of being a professional

Introduction

Change means modifying behaviour, a common preoccupation for professionals and their managers. There is a large literature on change management in health care, with diverse theories and models, and yet sustained quality improvement (QI) seems to be one of the most difficult tasks for health systems to achieve. The few examples of successful and sustained large-scale QI collaborations are counterbalanced by many of limited, or no, efficacy.

Unreliable care – the gap between desired and actual practice, expressed as the proportion of errors to total opportunities for error – is very common. Box 16.1 shows how reliability of health care compares with civil aviation.

Box 16.1 **Reliability of health care compared to civil aviation**

Activity	Reliability rate	Number of episodes producing 10 errors
Civil aviation	10^{-6}	1 million
Anaesthesia, blood transfusion	10^{-4}	10 000
Rest of health care	10^{-2}	100

Reliability improvement is particularly challenging in acute and emergency care. Acutely ill patients are characterized by the severity and diagnostic uncertainty of their illness, and their rapidly

changing physical states; their care must be maintained for long periods of time – many days or weeks – often delivered out-of-hours, with multiple transitions between teams and geographical areas, and lapses in communication. Process control, which is essential for reliability improvement, is difficult to maintain in these circumstances.

Sepsis is the most lethal and complex disorder to affect acutely ill patients. In October 2002, the Surviving Sepsis Campaign was launched to reduce mortality from sepsis by identifying, promoting and standardizing best practice worldwide. Like all QI collaboratives, this means changing clinical behaviour across diverse health systems in different countries. In this chapter, we will examine barriers to, and methods of, change management, with particular reference to acute care and sepsis.

Barriers and facilitators for changing behaviour

Change is a requirement for progress and improvement, but does not equate to it. Most healthcare workers have at some point been encouraged to adopt new interventions, which subsequently failed to demonstrate benefit or were found to cause harm, and a degree of scepticism may be appropriate. Frequent 'top-down' government initiatives implemented locally by management teams are unlikely to be adopted with enthusiasm by front-line staff confronting the daily complexities of patient care. The effort required for QI is often not recognized and rewarded in the same way as other research interventions, and the research methodologies are perceived as less robust. It is therefore more difficult to demonstrate and disseminate the success of QI initiatives, and they may require more effort to implement.

'Change' will only result in improvement if it is approached in a systematic and integrated manner, considering the intervention itself; the individuals who will implement it; the social, cultural and organisational factors in the system and the tools available to assess performance and outcomes. Understanding the reasons for failure to deliver high-reliability care is essential knowledge in designing improvement projects.

Interventions: guidelines and bundles

Evidence-based medicine provides an important framework for guideline development, but it does not in itself remove the need

ABC of Sepsis. Edited by Ron Daniels and Tim Nutbeam. © 2010 by Blackwell Publishing, ISBN: 978-1-4501-8194-5.

to make judgements. An important question for clinicians is 'what sort of evidence do you need to change your practice?'

The grading of recommendations assessment, development and evaluation (GRADE) system makes it easier to consider separately the strength of evidence and the strength of the recommendation, an important distinction for QI work where it may be impossible to conduct randomized controlled trials of established treatments (for example, timing of antibiotics for septic shock, rationing access to intensive care units or hand hygiene). When evidence is weak or conflicting, recommendations can nonetheless be made, aided by the availability of consensus expert opinion. Performed properly using formal techniques, this can show whether experts are in agreement, polarized, or in equipoise. This makes it easier to issue authoritative recommendations to clinicians, as well as to identify interventions that require further research.

Given the relative lack of impact of guidelines on clinical practice and the difficulty of operationalizing large numbers of recommendations, QI groups are starting to use care 'bundles' in an attempt to improve implementation. The principles of creating care bundles are described in Box 16.2. First proposed by the Institute for Healthcare Improvement (IHI), bundles have been adopted by the Joint Commission in the United States and the National Health Service in the United Kingdom, and are currently being evaluated by the Surviving Sepsis Campaign (Box 16.3). Advantages of bundling include the enforcement of best practice through uniformity and reducing complexity. Potential disadvantages include disagreements about component elements, concerns over legal implications of failure to implement and the absence of evidence at present that bundling is effective – though this may be forthcoming.

Box 16.2 **Principles of bundling**

- Include high-evidence or strong recommendation interventions
- Include interventions which gap analyses have shown are performed unreliably
- Minimize the number of components
- Interventions should share same time and location
- Aim to complete all elements

Box 16.3 **Severe Sepsis Resuscitation Bundle**

Within six hours of first identifying severe sepsis or septic shock, complete the following tasks:

- Measure serum lactate
- Obtain blood cultures before antibiotic administration
- Give broad-spectrum antibiotics in <3 hours for Emergency Department (ED) admissions and <1 hour for non-ED admissions

In the event of hypotension and/or a serum lactate >4 mmol/l:

- Deliver an initial minimum of 20 ml/kg of crystalloid or equivalent volume of colloid
- Use vasopressors for hypotension not responding to initial fluid resuscitation to maintain mean arterial pressure (MAP) >65 mmHg

---

In the event of persistent hypotension despite fluid resuscitation and/or lactate >4 mmol/l:

- Achieve a central venous pressure (CVP) of ≥8 mmHg
- Achieve a central venous oxygen saturation (ScvO$_2$) ≥70% or mixed venous oxygen saturation (SvO$_2$) ≥65%

Individuals

Changing the behaviour of people, and thus of whole systems, takes courage, persistence, willingness to learn from others and leadership from in front. It also helps if, as Truman said, you do not care who gets the credit for success. This is not just an issue for healthcare professionals: patients also need to be empowered as partners in improving their own outcomes. Some of the more common human factors contributing to low reliability care are given in Table 16.1. Barriers to implementing best practice vary widely as individuals' attitudes and behaviour vary. Competence does not equate to excellence and capacity does not equal delivery, and the gaps between each are more common than deficits in knowledge. Competence-based training is important in defining educational outcomes, but it needs to be accompanied by a strong focus on attitudes and behaviours to ensure that excellence becomes a habit.

The system: social and organizational factors

Systems are only as good as the individuals within them; structures and traditions can enhance or impede individual effort. The organizational structure should, therefore, be based on clear strategic aims. Absence of strategic direction or front-line leadership results in loss of discipline. Insufficient or unsatisfactory resources are a common problem, particularly when management success is measured in terms of cost containment or throughput targets rather

Table 16.1 Individual barriers to changing behaviour.

Component	Example
Dissociation in time of process failure from subsequent associated adverse event	Central venous catheter bacteraemias
Underestimation of importance or frequency of adverse event	Hypokalaemia in acutely ill patients
Low expectations: tolerance of poor standards as the norm	Communication failures. Hygiene failures. Reluctance to give, or receive, criticism
Dysfunctional attitudes and professionalism	'Not my job' syndrome. Emotional dissociation from patient-centred outcomes; burnout
Roles, responsibilities, prestige and power	Lack of empowerment; rigid demarcation of roles; steep hierarchies; fear of blame
Reluctance to standardize care and limit professional autonomy	Protocol deviations without evident reason; suboptimal teamworking
Lack of knowledge	Professional isolation; lack of continuing training; competence-excellence gap
Workload	Multitasking; too many priorities; lack of support

than reliability. Resources must be made available for all aspects of reliability improvement, including staff development. James Reason has described 'blaming front line individuals, denying the existence of systemic error provoking weaknesses, and the blinkered pursuit of productive and financial indicators' as features of the vulnerable systems syndrome.

Vertical hierarchies and professional 'silos' inhibit effective communication and transdisciplinary learning, a particular problem for acutely ill patients whose journey through the healthcare system crosses speciality and geographical boundaries. The differing authority and power of doctors, nurses and patients make it difficult in some cultures to challenge and correct errors, a major problem in acute care where system tolerances may be low. Team working means some loss of professional autonomy, but this is not incompatible with taking personal responsibility, having pride in one's work and leadership. Good role models and effective opinion leaders are essential in developing an organization which is patient focused, transparent, reflective, self-critical, supportive and forward looking.

Tools, methods and metrics for improvement

Tools

There is no single ideal method or tool for implementing and sustaining changes in clinical practice. Multifaceted interventions may be no more effective than properly applied single interventions. Some interventions are necessarily multifaceted, for example, rapid response (medical emergency or outreach) teams, in which case the content of the intervention should be made explicit.

Mortality and morbidity meetings are of limited use without measurable actions and objectives. Gap analyses can provide convincing evidence of the need for QI: clinicians consistently overestimate their adherence to best practice.

Plan-Do-Study-Act (PDSA) cycles were developed as a method for enabling small-scale rapid change evaluations to grow into systems-wide performance improvement. Like care bundles, systematic evaluations of efficacy are lacking, but the technique has face validity as a useful tool for initiating change at a local level.

Clinical decision support is most effective if it is provided at the point of care and incorporated in routine workplace activities. Computerized reminders for therapies or laboratory investigations are most helpful if they reduce clinical work, for example, by providing automated prescriptions for validation. Requesting documentation of the reasons for deviating from established guidelines also improves compliance.

Educational interventions such as passive distribution of materials, small group teaching and educational outreach or academic detailing have limited effects unless accompanied by specific action plans or reinforcement. Reliability improvement needs to be built into life-long learning, for example, by integrating best practice guidelines with national and international competency-based training programmes across disciplines.

Methods, metrics and ethics

QI research should start with a research question and a literature review. The intervention may target efficacy, effectiveness, efficiency or implementation strategy. Baseline data are essential for determining event rates. It is important to minimize the burden of data collection, as QI research may need to be conducted over long periods with minimal resources. Existing clinical databases may be used or adapted to assess the stability of pre-intervention baseline event rates, the effect of the intervention and post-intervention sustainability.

Two important methodological challenges are whether to monitor process or outcome and to identify a suitable control group. Process monitoring is more empowering (the participants can do something about it) and data collection is immediate; outcomes are more important to patients, but data collection is delayed, and the link between process and outcome may be complex. There is substantial uncertainty and diversity at present about the institutional review and safety monitoring requirements of QI activities. Indeed, there is a view that QI should not be classified as research at all, on the basis that all clinicians have a duty to review and improve their clinical care. One consensus statement on this issue proposes that QI should not require institutional review for ethical approval. It is important, however, for those engaged in QI activities to appreciate that the perceived need for consent, or intent to publish, are not sufficient criteria to decide on whether ethical approval is needed. Given the spectrum of QI studies from multi-centre cluster randomized studies to small local initiatives implementing best practices, consultation with an institutional review board is a safe option.

A practical approach

QI research is challenging precisely because it involves changing behaviour. We have provided a synopsis of the steps required in Box 16.4, based on our experiences and that of colleagues. The first two steps are perhaps the most important to understand the current 'environment' and to gather broad support for the project. Involvement and support of front-line colleagues is essential; audit and gap analysis can be undertaken by trainees as a local project, across disciplines if appropriate. This should be accompanied by a survey of current behaviour and barriers to change. The 'new' behaviour is the intervention, which requires consideration of all the components in the patient journey where the intervention could be applied. Improvement tools should be as simple as possible, and designed with the active involvement of those who will use them. Clarify common objectives: what will success look like and how will you know if the project has succeeded? Finally, take a long-term view: demonstrable success must be embedded in sustained improvement through long-term changes in behaviour.

Box 16.4 **Planning an improvement project**

1. Evaluate:
  a. The behaviour to change: reliability improvement
  b. The literature: best practice
  c. The environment:
    i. Audit and gap analysis (baseline data)
    ii. Current knowledge, barriers to change and culture
  d. The intervention: content, and mode of delivery
  e. The need for institutional or ethics review

2. Engage: those who have greatest impact on care

    a. Establish QI collaborative: stakeholders may include clinicians, managers, patients

    b. Identify local project leaders ('champions') in participating clinical areas

3. Educate:

    a. Develop improvement tools: educational materials, prompts, reminders, check lists

    b. Test and refine tools in small steps (Plan-Do-Study-Act (PDSA) cycles)

    c. Present project and background materials (nurse handovers, staff meetings, hospital Board)

4. Execute: implement effective behaviour change strategies

    a. Introduce improvement tools according to planned strategy

    b. Empower front-line staff to monitor compliance

5. Evaluate:

    a. Documentation of compliance (process monitoring)

    b. Impact on outcomes (if part of methodology)

    c. Revise according to user feedback (multiple PDSA cycles)

6. Embed: improvement tools in routine practice to sustain long-term

Further reading

Bero LA, Grilli R, Grimshaw JM, Harvey A, Oxman AD & Thomson MA, The Cochrane Effective Practice and Organization of Care Review Group. Closing the gap between research and practice: an overview of systematic reviews of interventions to promote the implementation of research findings. *British Medical Journal* 1998; **317** (7156): 465–468.

Bion JF & Heffner J. Improving hospital safety for acutely ill patients. A lancet quintet. I: current challenges in the care of the acutely ill patient. *Lancet* 2004; **363**: 970–977.

Brown CA & Lilford RJ. The stepped wedge trial design: a systematic review. *BMC Medical Research Methodology* 2006; **6**: 54; doi:10.1186/1471-2288-6-54.

Brunkhorst FM, Engel C, Jaschinsky U et al., the German Competence Network Sepsis (SepNe). Treatment of severe sepsis and septic shock in Germany: the gap between perception and practice – results from the german prevalence study. *Infection* 2005; **33** (Suppl 1): 49.

Cabana MD, Rand CS, Powe NR et al. Why don't physicians follow clinical practice guidelines? A framework for improvement. *The Journal of the American Medical Association* 1999; **282** (15): 1458–1465.

Cook DJ, Montori VM, McMullin JP, Finfer SR & Rocker GM. Improving patients' safety locally: changing clinician behaviour. *Lancet* 2004; **363**: 1224–1230.

Curtis RJ, Cook DJ, Wall RJ et al. Intensive care unit quality improvement: a 'how-to' guide for the interdisciplinary team. *Critical Care Medicine* 2006; **34**: 211–218.

Dellinger RP, Levy MM, Carlet JM et al. Surviving Sepsis Campaign: international guidelines for management of severe sepsis and septic shock: 2008. Special Article. *Critical Care Medicine* 2008; **36** (1): 296–327.

Eccles M, Grimshaw J, Campbell M & Ramsay C. Research designs for studies evaluating the effectiveness of change and improvement strategies *Quality and Safety in Health Care* 2003; **12**: 47–52; doi:10.1136/qhc.12.1.47.

GRADE Working Group. Grading quality of evidence and strength of recommendations. *British Medical Journal* 2004; **328**: 1490–1498.

Grimshaw JM, Thomas RE, MacLennan G et al. Effectiveness and efficiency of guideline dissemination and implementation strategies. *Health Technology Assessment* 2004; **8** (6): 1–72.

Grol R, Berwick DM & Wensing M. On the trail of quality and safety in health care. *British Medical Journal* 2008; **336**: 74–76; doi:10.1136/bmj.39413.486944.AD.

http://www.clean-safe-care.nhs.uk/. NHS website devoted to the reduction of healthcare-associated infection, accessed 2008.

http://www.survivingsepsis.org/. Website of the international Surviving Sepsis Campaign, accessed 2008.

Institute of Medicine. Committee on Quality of Health Care in America. *Crossing the Quality Chasm: A New Health System for the 21st Century*. National Academy Press, Washington, DC, 2001.

Lynn J, Baily M, Bottrell M et al. The ethics of using quality improvement methods in health care. *Annals of Internal Medicine* 2007; **146**: 666–673.

McGlynn EA, Asch SM, Adams J, Keesey J, Hicks J, DeCristofaro A & Kerr EA The quality of health care delivered to adults in the USA. *New England Journal of Medicine* 2003; **348**: 2635–2645.

Neuhauser D & Diaz M. Quality improvement research: are randomised trials necessary? *Quality and Safety in Health Care* 2007; **16**: 77–80; doi:10.1136/qshc.2006.021584.

Pronovost PJ, Berenholtz SM, Goeschel CA et al. Creating high reliability in health care organizations. *Health Services Research* 2006; **41** (4p2): 1599–1617; doi:10.1111/j.1475-6773.2006.00567.x.

Pronovost P, Needham D, Berenholtz S et al. An intervention to decrease catheter-related bloodstream infections in the ICU. *New England Journal of Medicine* 2006; **355** (26): 2725–2732.

Pronovost P & Wachter R. Proposed standards for quality improvement research and publication: one step forward and two steps back. *Quality and Safety in Health Care* 2006; **15**: 152–153; doi:10.1136/qshc.2006.018432.

Raising the Bar with Bundles: Treating patients with an all-or-nothing standard. *Joint Commission Perspectives on Patient Safety* 2006; **6** (4): 5–6.

Reason JT, Carthey J & de Leval MR. Diagnosing "vulnerable system syndrome": an essential prerequisite to effective risk management. *Quality in Health Care* 2001; **10**: ii21–ii25.

Rubenfeld DG. Surrogate measures of patient-centered outcomes in critical care. In: Sibbald WS & Bion JF, eds. *Evaluating Critical Care: Using Health Services Research to Improve Quality*. Springer, Berlin, 2001: 23–40.

Tan JA, Naik VN & Lingard L. Exploring obstacles to proper timing of prophylactic antibiotics for surgical site infections. *Quality and Safety in Health Care* 2006; **15**: 32–38; doi:10.1136/qshc.2004.012534.

The CoBaTrICE Collaboration. consensus development of an international competency-based training programme in Intensive Care Medicine. *Intensive Care Medicine* 2006; **32**: 1371–1383.

Thor J, Lundberg J, Ask J, Olsson J, Carli C, Härenstam KP & Brommels M. Application of statistical process control in healthcare improvement: systematic review. *Quality and Safety in Health Care* 2007; **16**: 387–399; doi:10.1136/qshc.2006.022194.

Index

Page numbers in *italics* represent figures, those in **bold** represent tables.